The Camp Health Manual

The Camp Health Manual
David Goldring, M.D. and J. Neal Middelkamp, M.D.

American Camping Association
Martinsville, Indiana

Disclaimer

The information and advice set forth in this manual should be very carefully reviewed in each particular situation and is intended only as a guide for doctors and nurses.

American Camping Association, Inc., hereby disclaims any and all responsibility or liability, which may be asserted or claimed arising from or claimed to have arisen from reliance upon the contents set forth in this manual by doctors, nurses, or others.

ISBN 0-87603-072-X

Published by the American Camping Association
Martinsville, Indiana 46151-7902

©1984, American Camping Association
All Rights Reserved
Printed in the United States of America

To Evie and S., N., P., M., and J.

and

To Lois and S., S., S., S., J., S., and G.

TABLE OF CONTENTS

    Preface xi
    Acknowledgements xiii
I.   CAMP STANDARDS 1
II. THE INFIRMARY 11
III. INFIRMARY SUPPLIES 20
IV. COMMON MEDICAL AND SURGICAL PROBLEMS 27
V.   PSYCHIATRIC DISORDERS 41
VI. CAMPING AND THE HANDICAPPED CHILD 57
VII. EAR, NOSE, THROAT, AND CHEST PROBLEMS 67
VIII. SKIN PROBLEMS 73
IX. ALLERGIC DISORDERS 82
X.   EYE INJURY AND INFECTIONS 85
XI. BITES BY SNAKES, ANIMALS, AND SPIDERS 90
XII. THE ROLE OF THE CAMP HEALTH SUPERVISOR
      IN EMERGENCIES 102
    Appendix I 121
    Appendix II 150

FOREWORD

The health and safety of the child at camp has always been the first concern of both the parent and the camp director. The *Camp Physician's Manual*, written by a prominent pediatrician with long experience as a camp doctor, is of inestimable value to the camp director who carries this heavy responsibility.

The need for such a book has long been felt. This is, I believe, the first complete recording of medical and health service in a camp setting. It covers every aspect of health care for campers and staff, from setting up a health center to waterfront safety, and from refrigeration to sanitation—in other words, the total range of health responsibility in camping.

The book is written in an interesting style with excellent understanding and insight into the special situation that exists in a camp setting. The material is completely professional and scientific, and it will be of great value and service to the camp director, nurse, and doctor.

I congratulate Dr. Goldring on a most significant contribution to the literature of camping, and I highly recommend his book to the camping profession.

Stanley J. Michaels
Past President
American Camping Association

EDITOR'S NOTE: The Camp Physician's Manual, published in 1967 and written by Dr. David Goldring served for many years as the best material in the field of health care in summer camps. The foreword by Stanley J. Michaels is as pertinent to the new book.

PREFACE

During the summers of the late fifties and early sixties my family and I spent four weeks at a boys' camp, where I served as camp physician. We had wonderful times in the camp, because the medical responsibilities were not too taxing nor time-consuming, and the swimming and fishing were great.

As a pediatrician, I had no qualms about assuming the responsibilities of a camp doctor, because I was reasonably certain that the demands of the job would be no more difficult than that of the pediatric emergency room. The work was not difficult, and the medical and surgical problems were relatively minor. I realized, however, that a physician not trained as a pediatrician would not be acquainted with common pediatric medical problems and would need an on-the-spot reference book as a guide in diagnosis, drug dosage, and therapy of the sick campers.

During that period, I gradually learned what role the physician plays in this small community—the summer camp—and realized that a camp doctor will do a much more effective job if he comes to camp oriented in the philosophy of camping, the physical composition and the administrative structure of a camp, and with a sensitivity to the interrelationships of the camper, counselor, camp director, and parents.

I have held numerous briefing sessions with physicians who were planning to spend several weeks as a camp doctor, because it became known around the medical center that I had camping experience. Often, I was asked if a book or other reading material were available which dealt with the duties and responsibilities of a camp physician. Since I could not find a guide book on this subject, I decided to prepare a manual which was published in 1967.

The information in that manual was organized so that each minor or major medical problem was treated in a realistic manner. The counselor's role as a first aid person was briefly described. The nurse's duties in the management of the sick camper were outlined. I tried to present the material so that it would be of help in the management of medical and surgical problems by the camp counselor, camp director, or the camp nurse, as well as the resident or practicing physician, the internist, pediatrician, surgeon, ophthalmologist, obstetrician, or the person in general practice who was going to spend a portion of the summer as a camp physician.

When the American Camping Association asked whether I would be interested in updating the manual, after some deliberation, I decided to do so.

I envisioned that the revisions would not have to be major, but a number of changes were certainly needed. The field of pediatrics has undergone major changes in the last 15 years so that we have now recognized subspecialties in Pediatrics. With this in mind, I invited Dr.

Barbara Herjanic, Associate Professor in Pediatrics and Psychiatry and staff psychiatrist at St. Louis Children's Hospital, to write the chapter on psychological disorders. Dr. J. Neal Middelkamp, Professor of Pediatrics on our staff, collaborated with me to write the sections on common surgical and medical problems, eye injuries and infections, and ear, nose, and throat problems. Dr. Middelkamp also revised Appendix I which is a description of various diseases in outline form as well as the chapter on snake, animal, and spider bites. Dr. Donald B. Strominger was Clinical Professor of Pediatrics whose specialty was allergy, prepared the chapter on allergic problems, and Dr. Tom W. Cooper, Instructor in Dermatology, prepared the chapter on skin problems. I should like to express my thanks to all of the above.

David Goldring
November 1, 1982

ACKNOWLEDGEMENTS

We wish to express our thanks for the critical review of the chapter on ear, nose, and throat problems by Dr. Kenneth Faw, formerly Assistant Professor of Otolaryngolgy; the chapter on eye problems by Dr. James Miller, formerly Professor of Ophthalmology; and the section on surgical problems by Dr. Jessie Ternberg, Professor of Surgery, all members of the faculty of Washington University School of Medicine and the St. Louis Children's Hospital.

We wish to express our sincere appreciation to Lorraine Vandersteen for typing the manuscript and to Donna Cherry, Kim Kendall, and Aileen Derhake for the final typing of the book.

Finally, we wish to say an extra special thank you to our wives, Evie and Lois, for their encouragement during the preparation of this book.

D. G., J. N. M.

The photographs in this book were taken at Camp Riley, Bradford Woods, Martinsville, Indiana.

Chapter I

CAMP STANDARDS

The camp Health Supervisor* should be knowledgeable about the overall organization, sanitation, and safety regulations of a camp, so that his/her judgement and operating procedure will be sound and sensible in the event of illness or accident caused by a breakdown in any of the above-mentioned areas. Such a breakdown may jeopardize the health and safety of the entire camp. For example, activities may be completely disrupted by a precipitous outbreak of gastroenteritis or streptococcal throat infection. In such emergencies, a Health Supervisor who understands the organization, sanitation facilities, and safety regulations of a camp will engender a feeling of confidence in his/her professional ability, judgement, and course of action.

The inexperienced camp Health Supervisor can quickly learn about the above by reviewing *Camp Standards with Interpretations* (generally known as "The Standards Book") which is published by the American Camping Association (ACA). We should like to emphasize that this is essential reading in the preparation and orientation of a physician or nurse who has never been a camp Health Supervisor. We shall briefly review some of the aspects covered in the above publication, which should give the prospective Health Supervisor a flavor of the contents of the publication.

Nature and Location of Camp

In the introduction to the health care Standards, the ACA Standards Book points out that camps vary widely both in their locations and the availability of dependable community health care services, as well as in the daily in-camp health care needs of the clientele. The ACA Camp Standards are designed to encourage camps to develop responsible health care systems that are appropriate to their particular settings. Obviously, the physician is key counsel to the camp administration in this process.

ACA points out four variables which should be considered in determining health care recommendations:

1. Strenuousness of the camp program activities.
2. Remoteness of the camp or program group from family, with whom health care decisions can be shared.
3. Remoteness of the camp or program group from medical assistance.
4. Special health care needs of participants.

---

*In this volume where a responsibility is one that may be carried out by a physician or a nurse under standing orders from the camp physician, the term Health Supervisor is used.

Often, though the camp may be located with access to good community medical services, groups from the camp may go "trip camping" in very remote areas. This requires that the camp Health Supervisor play a very active role in the preparation of the trip camping staff to handle routine health care needs as well as emergencies on the trip.

In general, the ACA Standards are organized around general areas of camp administration, and each area contains some elements of special interest to the physician. Throughout the Standards there are those which require special considerations for persons with special health care needs such as physical disabilities, diabetes, epilepsy, or mental retardation.

Site Standards

The site Standards cover the characteristics of site and facilities and the procedures necessary to utilize and protect them. Included are such things as the size, spaciousness, and exits associated with sleeping units; ratios of toilets, bathing, and hand washing facilities to users; fire protection for all buildings; availability of laundry services, if needed; and, of course, use of approved water supplies and sewage disposal systems.

Administration Standards

Included in the administration area are a host of Standards covering goals, plans, arrangements, policies, and procedures governing the general camp operation. Of particular interest to the camp physician would be those addressing information collected on all campers and staff, policies governing release of information and provision of any professional therapy, the camp's risk management plan, insurance coverages, sanitation, handling and storage of hazardous equipment and materials, emergency procedures, and safety regulations related particularly to transportation.

Food Service Standards

For camps which store and/or serve food, there are Standards of particular importance in health care. Standards regarding the storage and handling of food and the cleanliness of the food preparation area and utensils are of particular significance. Standards recommend that the meals be planned or approved by a nutritionist and/or dietitian. The camp Health Supervisor will want to work closely with this person, particularly for those individuals in camp which have special dietary needs.

Health Care Standards

The health care Standards address such things as the precamp comprehensive health examination by a licensed physician. The camp physician should help the camp administration design information for the examining physicians which will communicate the nature of the camp experience for which the camper is being examined, particularly if the camp will likely create physical and emotional stresses which are much different from those at home, school, or work.

Other health care Standards include the collection of an up-to-date health history from parents of minors or adults in camp, the conduct of initial health screening by a health care professional, required record-keeping systems in camp and after camp, the first aid preparation of camp staff, characteristics of a camp infirmary, and special personnel and procedural requirements for camps serving persons with special health care needs.

A key responsibility of the camp physician is the development and authorization for use of standing orders. The ACA Standards state that all staff who provide any level of health care should be furnished appropriate specific written procedures, supplies, and equipment and that they be given training in their use. This is to include the utilization of standing orders signed annually by the camp physician which cover: 1) the initial health screening (if not conducted by the camp physician), 2) routine health care and medical treatment (other than that rendered by the camp physician), 3) first aid procedures and kit contents (many use the recommendations of the American Red Cross in this area, except for the specialized tripping situations mentioned earlier), and 4) any health education which is a part of the camp program.

Personnel Standards

The personnel Standards include such things as recommendations for the age, education, and experience qualifications of various staff members. They also include ratios of staff to campers and various administrative practices such as contracts, job descriptions, personnel policies, etc. Of particular interest to the camp Health Supervisor is the precamp and in-service training received by the camp staff. The Health Supervisor will want to be an active part of this training process as it relates to health care responsibilities, as the camp counselor is often the key in the early identification of problems which need referral, as well as the person involved in initial first aid treatment. Also, the Health Supervisor is responsible for the health care of staff during the camp season, as well as for campers. Staff often present some unique health care problems, particularly in the resident camp setting which is often a more fatiguing experience, physically and emotionally, than other types of employment.

Program Standards

The program Standards address the variety of experiences the camp program should provide for campers and some elements of the conduct of a camp community. ACA has some additional Standards which apply to all camp activities which contain "controlled physical risk." These Standards cover written operating procedures and safety regulations, qualified staff, and appropriate equipment. Leaders are also to be provided with information regarding special health care needs of participants and oriented to any potential medical emergencies which might relate specifically to the activity in question.

Additionally, some of the more common camp activities which contain elements of "controlled risk" have their own sets of supplemental Standards. These include: aquatics, travel camping, tripping, and horseback riding.

Ideally, all resident camps should have a resident physician and a registered nurse on the staff. This is not possible in the majority of camps in the United States.

The camp physician is often a physician in the local town near the camp who is retained by the camp to serve the camp community. As part of that responsibility, the camp physician:

1. Reviews the Camp Health Plan, including:

a. First aid in camp program
b. Emergency medical care, including appropriate emergency transportation
c. Arrangements for care by the physician and/or admittance to the nearest hospital
d. Daily medical care (that requiring state-approved health care providers)
e. Routine health care for campers and staff
f. Supervision of camp health and sanitation practices; and
g. Arrangements for professional therapy (when provided)

2. Prepares the standing orders for the camp nurse.
3. Prepares a list of medications recommended for the camp health service.
4. Reviews the health examination and health screening forms utilized by the camp. (See *Figures 1, 2,* and *3.*)
5. Serves as the admitting doctor for the local camp's hospital and often serves by being on call in the case of an emergency.

Where there is no camp physician in residence, the camp nurse assumes duties as the Health Supervisor.

It is important that there be a pre-camp conference and a close working relationship between the camp physician and the camp nurse(s).

Most states require in-state licensing of physicians and registered nurses, even though the period of residence is 2-8 weeks. Laws governing licenses or practice vary from state to state, and it is advisable for the camp director, nurses, and physician to check with the particular state

Figure 1
Camp Health History and Examination Form

CAMP HEALTH HISTORY AND EXAMINATION FORM FM08
FOR CHILDREN, YOUTH AND ADULTS
Developed by
American Camping Association, Inc., in consultation with
The American Medical Association and the American Academy of Pediatrics

RETURN TO:

By _____ (Date)

This side to be filled in by parents/guardian of minors or by adult campers/staff members themselves.

Name _____ Birth Date _____ Sex _____ Age _____
       Last   First   Initial
Parent or Guardian (or Spouse) _____ Phone _____
                                                                                                          Area/Number
  Home Address _____
                 Street & Number   City   State   Zip Code
  Business Address _____ Phone _____
                Street & Number City   State   Zip Code   Area/Number

Second Parent or Guardian or Emergency Contact: _____
  Home Address _____ Phone _____
                Street & Number City   State   Zip Code   Area/Number
  Business Address _____ Phone _____
                Street & Number City   State   Zip Code   Area/Number

If not available in an emergency, notify:
  Name _____ Phone _____
                                                                           Area/Number
  Address _____
           Street & Number   City   State   Zip Code

Health History: *(Check—giving approximate dates)*   **Allergies**

		Diseases		
Frequent Ear Infections	_____	Mononucleosis _____	Hay Fever	_____
Heart Defect/Disease	_____		Ivy Poisoning, etc.	_____
Convulsions	_____	Chicken Pox _____	Insect Stings	_____
Diabetes	_____	Measles _____	Penicillin	_____
Bleeding/Clotting Disorders	_____	German Measles _____	Other Drugs	_____
Hypertension	_____	Mumps _____	Asthma	_____

Operations or serious injuries *(dates)*: _____
Disability or chronic or recurring illness: _____

Any specific activities to be encouraged or limited by physician's advice: _____

Dietary modifications. _____
Current medication *(send with instructions)*: _____
Other diseases or details of above: _____
Name of dentist/orthodontist: _____ Phone _____
                                                                                   Area/Number
Name of family physician: _____ Phone _____
                                                                                  Area/Number
Date of last physical examination: _____
Do you carry family medical/hospital insurance? _____ If so, indicate:
  Carrier: _____ Policy or Group # _____
Suggestions or health related information for camp personnel: _____

(For Female): Has this person menstruated? _____ If not, has she been told about it? _____
             If so, is her menstrual history normal? _____ Special Consideration: _____

Important—This Box Must be Completed for Attendance*

This health history is correct so far as I know, and the person herein described has permission to engage in all prescribed camp activities except as noted.

Emergency Authorization: I hereby give permission to the medical personnel selected by the camp director to order X-rays, routine tests and treatment for me/or my child, and in the event I cannot be reached in an emergency, I hereby give permission to the physician selected by the camp director to hospitalize, secure proper treatment for, and to order injection and/or anesthesia and/or surgery for me/or my child as named above. This form may be photocopied for use out of camp.

Signature of parent or guardian or adult camper/staffer _____
Witness: _____ Date _____
I also understand and agree to abide with the restrictions placed on my camp activities.
Signature of minor _____
                                            (OVER)

*If for religious reasons you cannot sign this, then the camp should be contacted for a legal waiver which must be signed for attendance.

Copyright 1983 by American Camping Association

Camper's Name _____ Date Examined _____ Cabin or Tent _____ Year _____

NOTE: Reverse side is identical to reverse side of health forms on pages 8 and 9.

Figure 1a
Camp Health History Form

**CAMP HEALTH HISTORY FORM FM 11
FOR CHILDREN, YOUTH AND ADULTS**

Developed by
American Camping Association, Inc., in consultation with
The American Medical Association and the American Academy of Pediatrics

RETURN TO:

By _____ (Date)

This side to be filled in by parents/guardian of minors or by adult campers/staff members themselves.

Name _____ (Last, First, Initial) Birth Date _____ Sex _____ Age _____
Parent or Guardian or Spouse _____ Phone _____ (Area, Number)
   Home Address _____ (Street & Number, City, State, Zip Code)
   Business Address _____ (Street & Number, City, State, Zip Code) Phone _____ (Area, Number)
Second Parent or Guardian or Emergency Contact: _____
   Home Address _____ (Street & Number, City, State, Zip Code) Phone _____ (Area, Number)
   Business Address _____ (Street & Number, City, State, Zip Code) Phone _____ (Area, Number)
If not available in an emergency, notify:
   Name _____ Phone _____ (Area, Number)
   Address _____ (Street & Number, City, State, Zip Code)

Health History: *(Check — giving approximate dates)*

			Allergies	
Frequent Ear Infections	____	Mononucleosis ____	Hay Fever	____
Heart Defect/Disease	____	**Diseases**	Ivy Poisoning, etc.	____
Convulsions	____	Chicken Pox ____	Insect Stings	____
Diabetes	____	Measles ____	Penicillin	____
Bleeding/Clotting Disorders	____	German Measles ____	Other Drugs	____
Hypertension	____	Mumps ____	Asthma	____

Operations or serious injuries *(dates):* _____
Disability or chronic or recurring illness: _____

Any specific activities to be encouraged or limited by physician's advice: _____

Dietary modifications: _____
Current medication *(send with instructions):* _____
Other diseases or details of above: _____
Name of dentist/orthodontist: _____ Phone _____ (Area Number)
Name of family physician: _____ Phone _____ (Area Number)
Date of last physical examination: _____
Do you carry family medical/hospital insurance? ____ If so, indicate:
   Carrier: _____ Policy or Group # _____
Suggestions or health related information for camp personnel: _____

(For Female): Has this person menstruated? ____ If not, has she been told about it? ____
   If so, is her menstrual history normal? ____ Special Consideration: _____

Important — This Box Must be Completed for Attendance*

This health history is correct so far as I know, and the person herein described has permission to engage in all prescribed camp activities except as noted.

Emergency Authorization: I hereby give permission to the medical personnel selected by the camp director to order X-rays, routine tests and treatment for me or my child, and in the event I cannot be reached in an emergency, I hereby give permission to the physician selected by the camp director to hospitalize, secure proper treatment for, and to order injection and/or anesthesia and/or surgery for me or my child as named above. This form may be photocopied for use out of camp.

Signature of parent or guardian or adult camper/staffer _____
Witness: _____ Date _____
I also understand and agree to abide with the restrictions placed on my camp activities.
Signature of minor _____
(OVER)

*If for religious reasons you cannot sign this, then the camp should be contacted for a legal waiver which must be signed for attendance.

Copyright 1983 by American Camping Association

Figure 1b
Camp Health History Form (reverse side)

IMMUNIZATION HISTORY

Required immunizations must be determined locally. Please record the date (month and year) of basic immunizations and most recent booster doses:

Vaccines	Year of Basic Immunization	Year of Last Booster
Diphtheria Pertussis (Whopping Cough)] DPT* Tetanus or	1 2 3	1 2
Tetanus Diphtheria] TD* or		
Tetanus		
Oral Polio (Sabin)* TOPV		
Injectable Polio (Salk)		
Measles (hard measles, red measles, Rubeola)		
Mumps		
Rubella (German measles, 3 day measles)		
Other		
Tuberculin test given _____ (most recent)		

FOR CAMP USE

In-camp Health Screening Record: *(Should conform to camp physician's written standing orders for camp screening. Note should be made of observations which are not already noted on the Health History.)*

ARRIVAL

Date _____ By _____
Observation Record
1. _____ Weight
2. _____ Temperature
3. Eyes: _____ Pain   _____ Drainage
            _____ Dislocation   _____ Pink
4. Nose: _____ Cold   _____ Nosebleeds
5. Ears: _____ Pain   _____ Drainage
6. Throat: _____ Red   _____ Sore
            _____ Cough
7. Teeth: _____ Cavities   _____ Pain
8. Posture: _____ Curvature of spine
9. Skin: _____ Presence of infection
10. Feet: _____ Athletes foot
            _____ Blisters   _____ Flat
11. Hair: _____ Lice
12. _____ Health history checked

DEPARTURE

Date _____ By _____
Observation Record
1. _____ Weight
2. _____ Temperature
3. Eyes: _____ Pain   _____ Drainage
            _____ Dislocation   _____ Pink
4. Nose: _____ Cold   _____ Nosebleeds
5. Ears: _____ Pain   _____ Drainage
6. Throat: _____ Red   _____ Sore
            _____ Cough
7. Teeth: _____ Cavities   _____ Pain
8. Posture: _____ Curvature of spine
9. Skin: _____ Presence of infection
10. Feet: _____ Athletes foot
            _____ Blisters   _____ Flat
11. Hair: _____ Lice

Record of any medications brought to camp.

_____

_____

_____

Medications returned to camper:

_____

_____

_____

Any other observations re: evidence of illness, disability, or communicable disease.

_____

_____

_____

Any follow-up recommended by person conducting health screening:

_____

_____

8/THE CAMP HEALTH MANUAL

Figure 2
Female Camp Health History and Examination Form

FEMALE CAMP HEALTH HISTORY AND EXAMINATION FORM FM 06
Developed by
American Camping Association, Inc.
in consultation with
The American Medical Association and the American Academy of Pediatrics

RETURN TO:

By _____

This is to be completed by parents, guardian of minors or by adult camper staff members themselves.

Name _____ Birthdate _____ Sex _____ Age _____
Parent or Guardian _____ Phone _____
Home Address _____
Business Address _____ Phone _____
Second Parent or Guardian _____
Home Address _____
Business Address _____ Phone _____
If not available in an emergency, notify
Name _____ Phone _____
Address _____

HEALTH HISTORY *(Check giving approximate dates)*
_____ Frequent Ear Infections
_____ Heart Defect, Disease
_____ Convulsions
_____ Diabetes
_____ Bleeding, Clotting Disorders
_____ Hypertension
_____ Mononucleosis
Diseases
_____ Chicken Pox
_____ Measles
_____ German Measles
_____ Mumps
Allergies
_____ Hay Fever
_____ Ivy Poisoning, etc.
_____ Insect Stings
_____ Penicillin
_____ Other Drugs
_____ Asthma

*If for religious reasons you cannot sign this, then the camp should be contacted for a legal waiver which must be signed for attendance.

Copyright 1983 by American Camping Association

Operations or serious injuries (dates) _____
Disabilities or chronic or recurring illness _____
Any specific activities to be encouraged or limited by physician's advice _____
Dietary modifications _____
Current medication (send with instructions) _____
Other diseases or details of above _____
Name of dentist/orthodontist _____ Phone _____
Name of family physician _____ Phone _____
Date of last physical examination _____ Do you carry family medical/hospital insurance? _____ If so, indicate
Carrier _____ Policy or Group # _____
Suggestions or health related information for camp personnel _____
Has this person menstruated? _____ If not, has she been told about it? _____ If so, is her menstrual history normal? _____

Important — This Box Must be Completed for Attendance*

This health history is correct so far as I know, and the person herein described has permission to engage in all prescribed camp activities except as noted. **Emergency Authorization:** I hereby give permission to the medical personnel selected by the camp director to order X-rays, routine tests and treatment for the health of my child, and in the event I cannot be reached in an emergency, I hereby give permission to the physician selected by the camp director to hospitalize, secure proper treatment for, and to order injection and/or anesthesia/surgery for my child as named above. This form may be photocopied for use out of camp.
Signature of parent or guardian or adult camper/staffer _____
Witness _____ Date _____
I also understand and agree to abide with the restrictions placed on my camp activities.
Signature of minor _____

IMMUNIZATION HISTORY

Required immunizations must be determined locally. Please record the dates (month and year) of basic immunizations and most recent doses:

Vaccines	Year of Basic Immunization	Year of Last Booster
Diphtheria ⎫	1	1
Pertussis (Whopping Cough) ⎬ DPT*	2	2
Tetanus ⎭	3	
or		
Tetanus ⎫ TD*		
Diphtheria ⎬		
or		
Tetanus		
Oral Polio (Sabin)* TOPV		
Injectable Polio (Salk)		
Measles (hard measles, red measles, Rubeola)		
Mumps		
Rubella (German measles, 3-day measles)		
Other		
Tuberculin test given _____ (most recent)		

Health Examination by Licensed Physician:
I have examined the above camp applicant within the past two years.
Date Examined: _____
In my opinion, the above's condition does _____ /does not _____ preclude his/her participation in an active camp program.

The applicant is under the care of a physician for the following condition(s): _____

Current treatment *(include current medications)*: _____

Explanation of any reported loss of consciousness, convulsions, concussion: _____

Does applicant have epilepsy? Yes _____ No _____
Does applicant have diabetes? Yes _____ No _____
Recommendations and Restrictions While at Camp:
Any treatment to be continued at camp: _____

Any medication to be administered at camp *(specific dosages)*: _____

Any medically prescribed meal plan or dietary restrictions: _____

Any allergies (food, drugs, plants & insects, etc.): _____

Additional Health Information: _____
Licensed Physician's Signature _____
Phone _____ Address _____

Date of Form Completion _____
*By _____

*Initial if completed by nurse or physician's assistant

(back)

CAMP STANDARDS/9

Figure 3
Male Camp Health History and Examination Form

board of medical examiners regarding these regulations in advance of the camp season.

If the camp physician does not wish to obtain a temporary license or if this is not feasible, medical coverage may be worked out in the following way. A physician from out-of-state will be able to diagnose illnesses and make recommendations to the camp director. He/she may also do physical examinations. He/she is not permitted to dispense medications or practice surgery. When a situation arises which he/she feels requires medical treatment beyond "first aid," an arrangement can be made to consult with a licensed physician near the camp who can see campers who require medication, surgical procedures, or hospitalization. Since most physicians spend about two weeks at camp, this procedure may be the simplest, most economic, and most effective arrangement.

Many camps arrange for medical coverage by working out an arrangement with a local physician to come into camp and do periodic physical examinations and act as consultant for the camp nurse for medical and surgical problems which are beyond the "first aid" stage.

The camp nurse should have a state license before beginning his/her duties. Some states permit the use of a Physician's Assistant as a camp nurse, provided he/she has a license to practice issued by the particular State Board and is operating under the supervision of a specific licensed physician.

Chapter II

THE INFIRMARY

Organization and Administration

Emergency Room

The emergency room floor should measure approximately 12 by 15 feet and should be well-lighted and ventilated. Ideally, a waiting room about the same size with chairs or benches should be available. There should be a closet for medications, which should be kept locked at all times when not in use, and the nurse and physician should be the only people with access to medications. There should be a washstand, an examination table, wastebaskets, an adequate overhead light, a lamp for spot-lighting (this light will be useful when suturing cuts, etc.), and benches and chairs. Bandages, tape, scissors, applicators, thermometers, tongue blades, etc., may be kept on an open-shelf cabinet. There may also be a table for a small sterilizer and a refrigerator for storing medications and as a source of ice cubes.

Hospital Rooms

The American Camping Association recommends one infirmary bed for every 35 campers. The hospitalization rooms may contain two to four beds, depending upon the size of the rooms. There should be a room with one to two beds for isolating campers who are suspected of having a contagious disease. The hospital rooms should have a reading light and a small table beside each bed. A clever nurse can improvise accessories such as disposable waste paper bags, bed tables, backrests, etc., which will add to the comfort of the sick campers. Of course, there should be toilet facilities, a shower, and washstands. These may be central or individual.

Records

The records of physical examinations, health histories, and screening of the staff and campers should be kept in the infirmary file, and from

Figure 4

Health Record Log

CAMP HEALTH RECORD

6

Date 8/10/83

Time	Name	Living Unit	Nature of Illness or Injury	Treatment or Disposition	Treated By
3:15	Joe Smith	Oak	T=98.6; mild redness of mucous membranes nose and throat	no swimming observe	JA
3:30	Tom Jones	West	Small, superficial abrasion over tibial tuberosity	washed w/soap and water; meran isolate (tincture) bandage	JA
4:30	Sue James	East	abdominal pain; no vomiting or diarrhea T=98.6 P.E.-neg.	observe to return	JA

these reports lists of individuals should be made which contain the following information:*

1. Campers who are allergic to specific foods and drugs;
2. Campers who are on special reducing diets at the request of the parents and/or the family physician;
3. Campers who are to have additional milk in the evening at the request of the parents and/or the family physician;
4. Campers who are receiving special daily medications, for example, antihistamine drugs, eye drops, anticonvulsant drugs, etc.
5. Also, special lists of campers who have physical handicaps such as a crippled extremity, deafness, blindness in one eye, orthodontic problems, psychological disorders (temper tantrums, bedwetting, sleepwalking, anxieties, etc.).

A daily log should be kept of the campers who are seen by the Health Supervisor because of illness or injury. The log should be bound with continuous entries on pre-numbered pages. Such a log has greater value in court than one which is not so organized. An example of a daily log may be seen in *Figure 4*. When a camper is placed upon medication which is to be given three to four times a day and remains ambulatory, a slip should be sent to the cabin counselor who will help to remind the camper to come to the infirmary for his medication. An example of such a form may be seen in *Figure 5*.

Some campers may have to be restricted from swimming because of external otitis media or a cut, etc. A "no swim" list should be posted daily so that the cabin counselor and the swimming staff know which campers are to be kept out of the water.

A complete record should be kept on hospitalized patients. A sample form is shown in *Figure 6*.

The campers are usually examined every two weeks during a camping season of eight weeks. This is a good practice, for it will help the camp Health Supervisor gain an impression of the general status of health in the camp. Also, not all campers come to see the Health Supervisor for colds, infected cuts, or insect bites. This will help prevent aggravation or complications of unreported injuries or infections. A form which may be used for these examinations is shown in *Figure 7*. In the event of an

---

*There are a number of campers who by history are known to be sensitive to certain drugs, foods, or pollens. This information is usually supplied by the parents and the family physician. The names of the campers who are sensitive to certain drugs should be kept for ready reference by the physician, and the name of any camper who is sensitive to certain foods should be given to his cabin counselor. There are usually a number of campers who are in the process of receiving desensitization therapy during camp (ragweed, house dust, etc.). The schedule for the weekly inoculations should be outlined by the physician for the camp nurse. Also, a number of campers may be taking oral therapy—usually antihistamines—and these drugs should be administered according to the instructions of the family physician. These lists should be posted for ready reference by the camp physician and nurse.

Figure 5

Infirmary Notice

Infirmary Notice

_____ is to report to the Infirmary after breakfast, lunch, dinner, and at bedtime for medication. Thank you for reminding him.

---

accident such as a fall from a horse, an auto accident, etc., a complete written record is vital so that information is available to the physician, camp director, parents, insurance company, or lawyers. A suggested form has been prepared by the American Camping Association and is shown in *Figure 8*.

The need and importance of such written records is obvious. Such records are important for a smoothly functioning infirmary and serve as a useful reference when there are inquiries from parents or the camp director.

The Health Supervisor should acquaint the counselors with special problems pertaining to campers. Occasionally a camper may have to be placed upon limited physical activity. The camper's counselor will be able to supervise this camper more effectively if the Health Supervisor alerts him to such limitations. If a camper is receiving medication at certain intervals, the counselor may be very helpful in getting the camper to the infirmary for the medication. A counselor may need guidance and support in dealing with campers who may have anxieties such as fear of the dark, night terrors, diet supervision, etc. The Health Supervisor should let the counselors know that he/she is available for help and consultation.

Letters should be sent to parents of campers admitted to the infirmary and also upon their discharge and return to full activity. This is an extremely important responsibility of the camp Health Supervisor. The campers may write to the parents about any mishap, and often their distorted accounts can be clarified by a prompt letter to the parents from the Health Supervisor. Carbon copies of such letters should be available so that the camp director is acquainted with this information, because he/she may receive phone calls from the parents inquiring about a mishap or illness.

If a camper is admitted to the infirmary, the cabin counselor should bring the camper's toilet articles, pajamas, robe, and slippers to the infirmary. The counselor should bring along any books the camper is reading and his stationery. A good camp nurse will try to keep the

Figure 6

Hospital Record

Name: John Jones
Cabin: 12
Counselor: Tom Smith

Date	Time	TPR	Meals	Fluids (ml)		Nurse's Remarks	Doctor's Notes
08-02-82	10:00 AM	101, 95, 20	Did not eat.	H₂O milk juice	240 200 60	Complains of sore throat. Asp. gr V. A.S.	P.E.: Moderate redness of pharynx, moderate anterior cervical adenopathy—face flushed. Moderately ill—admit to infirmary. Imp: acute pharyngitis. Treatment: (a) Aspirin, gr V (b) Force fluids (c) Observe D.G.
	12:00 NOON		Ate well.	juice	200		
	2:00 PM	99.4, 80, 20		milk gelatin	240 60	No complaints. A.S.	
	6:00 PM	98.6, 80, 20	Ate well.	H₂O juice milk	240 240	No complaints. A.S.	P.E. revealed no new findings; feels better; observe. D.G.
	10:00 PM	98.6, 80, 20		juice H₂O	200 200	No complaints. A.S.	
08-03-82	8:00 AM	98.6, 80, 20	Ate well.	milk juice	240 200	Feels fine. A.S.	Throat shows minimal redness; cervical adenopathy—about same; observe for one more day and then discharge. D.G.

Figure 7

CAMP HEALTH RECORD

(Individual — at Camp)

DEVELOPED AND APPROVED BY

AMERICAN CAMPING ASSOCIATION and AMERICAN ACADEMY OF PEDIATRICS

Camp Name

Name _____ Age _____ Sex _____

Entrance Date _____ Departure Date _____

| EXAMINATION | Departure By | IMPORTANT OBSERVATIONS TO FOLLOW WHILE AT CAMP |
Entrance By		
Height		
Weight		
Temperature		
Eyes		
Nose		
Ears		
Throat		
Teeth		
Posture		
Skin		
Feet		

Instructions and Report to Parents or Guardian: (Health Progress)

_____

_____

_____

_____

Signature _____

(OVER)

CAMPER'S NAME — Last, First, Initial

CABIN OR TENT

camper busy with reading matter, games, and craft work. The nurse may call upon the crafts counselor for help and suggestions. The campers are usually admitted because of relatively minor disorders and are kept in the infirmary at times as a precautionary measure. The campers will appreciate the added attention from the nurse. Good counselors will, of course, visit their campers and, when the illness is not contagious, they will encourage cabin-mates to visit the sick camper. A competent camp director will have indoctrinated counselors so that the sick camper is not forgotten during the illness. If this kind of sympathetic awareness is lacking in counselors, the Health Supervisor should tactfully call this to the attention of the camp director and counselors.

The camp Health Supervisor should make weekly rounds of the cabins, washhouses, and kitchen and look for areas which need attention or improvement. The rounds should include observation for any hazards about the camp grounds, such as boards with nails or broken glass. He/she should appraise general cleanliness and observe the adequacy of camper supervision as to appropriate clothing with changes in weather. It is very helpful in stimulating an awareness of camp health in the counseling staff if the Health Supervisor gives a weekly oral report at staff meetings about general health conditions in camp.

A physical examination or health screening at the conclusion of the camping season is advisable. The Health Supervisor can then write a note to the parents about those campers who need further medical attention upon their arrival home. The camper may have an upper respiratory infection, athlete's foot, a cut, or a large bruise. The parents will appreciate being notified by the Health Supervisor about even relatively minor disorders. This added bit of responsibility which a good camp Health Supervisor assumes will help cement the parents' feeling of confidence in the Health Supervisor, the camp, and the camp director.

A word of caution should be interjected here. The camp physician may not agree with the outline of therapy prescribed by the family physician (desensitization regimen, etc.). Obviously, it would be unwise to inform the parents about this unless there is flagrant medical mishandling of the camper. Also, it should be mentioned that calling the parents' attention to physical abnormalities unreported by the family physician should be done only after careful consideration. For example, a previously undetected heart murmur may be found by the camp physician. The camp physician should keep in mind that laboratory facilities for careful appraisal and examination are not available at camp. A carelessly written report will upset the parents and may disrupt the relationship between the family physician and the parents. If, in the sincere consideration of the Health Supervisor, a previously undiscovered abnormal finding is detected, this should, of course, be reported—but sound judgement and careful consideration should precede the written word.

Figure 8a
Accident Report Form

ACCIDENT REPORT FORM FM 01
Developed by
American Camping Association

Camp Name _____ Date _____

Address _____
                Street & Number   City   State   Zip Code

Name of Injured _____ Age ___ Sex ___ Camper ___ Staff ___ Visitor ___
                     Last   First   Middle

Address _____
                Street & Number   City   State   Zip Code

If Minor, Name of Parent/Guardian: _____

Address _____
                Street & Number   City   State   Zip Code

Names/Addresses of Witnesses (Attach signed statements as to incident.):

1. _____

2. _____

3. _____

Date of Accident _____ Hour _____ a.m.
                     (Day of Week)   (Month)   (Day)   (Year)   p.m.

Where occurred? (Specify location, including location of injured and witnesses. Use diagram to locate persons and objects.)

Describe accident in detail:

Was the injured participating in an activity at the time of the injury? _____ If so, what? _____

Any equipment involved in accident? _____

What could injured have done to prevent the injury? _____

Emergency procedures followed at time of accident: _____

By whom? _____

Submitted by _____ Position _____ Date _____

Copyright 1983 by American Camping Association

Figure 8b
Accident Report Form (reverse side)

Medical Report of Accident

Were parents notified? _____ In writing? _____ By phone? _____ Other _____
By whom? _____ When _____ _____
                                                                                                             Time   Date
Where was treatment given?   at camp _____ in camp health service _____ at doctor's office _____ in hospital _____
Treatment given at camp? _____ Where? _____
By whom? _____ Date _____
Treatment given _____
Was injured admitted to camp health service? _____ If so, when _____
Treatment given _____
Date released from health service _____
Released to: Camp activities _____ Home _____ Other _____
Treatment given elsewhere than camp? _____ Where? _____
By whom? _____ Date _____
Was injured admitted to hospital? _____ If so, which? _____
Where? _____ Date _____ Out-patient _____ In-patient _____
Name of physician in attendance _____
Date released from hospital _____
Released to: Camp _____ Health Service _____ Home _____ Other _____
Comments:

Signed _____ Position _____ Date _____
Insurance Claim/Report Submitted: Date
    1. _____ Parent's Insurance   By parent _____ By camp _____   _____
    2. _____ Camp Health Insurance   _____
    3. _____ Workman's Compensation   _____
    4. _____ Camp Liability Insurance   _____

Chapter III

INFIRMARY SUPPLIES

We have found the medications and supplies listed in *Table I* to be adequate for an eight-week camping season. These supplies are sufficient for the needs of approximately 300 campers, 40 counselors, and 20 support staff members.

The supplies listed in *Table I* are for camps which have a resident physician. Unfortunately, most camps do not have a camp physician. Since a nurse cannot dispense drugs which require a prescription by a physician, we have placed an asterisk before the supplies which require a prescription. The only exceptions are glucose and saline for intravenous administration on page 24. Adrenalin may be given by the nurse without a doctor's orders in the event of a life-threatening situation such as an anaphylactic reaction after a desensitization shot given by the nurse or a severe injury or burn where immediate parenteral fluids may be life-saving until the camper can be transported to a hospital. It might be more convenient for the camp without a resident physician to have all of these drugs. If a physician in a community close to camp is used and he/she prescribes drugs, it would be much more convenient for the nurse to dispense these drugs rather than purchasing the drugs in pharmacies in a community close to camp.

It is the responsibility of the nurse to take a careful inventory of the supplies at the start of the camping season. He/she should also keep a record of medications and supplies ordered. Finally, at the end of the camping season, another inventory should be taken, and on this should be noted the supplies and medications which will be needed for the next year.

It should be obvious that a good nurse will keep the medications and supplies well organized and easily accessible. The medications should be kept in locked closets and the keys should be available only to the nurse and physician.

The nurse is also responsible for having the supplies which require sterilization (gloves, suture tray, instruments) always ready for use.

Medicine should not be kept in the cabins. If a camper is upon special daily medication, such as antihistamine drugs, these should be kept in the infirmary, and the camper should come to the infirmary to take his medicine. In this way the nurse and physician will know that the camper is taking his medications.

Table I

Medications and Supplies

Antimicrobial Drugs Including Ophthalmics

*Amoxicillin caps 250 mg	1,000
caps 500 mg	500
Bacitracin Ointment 500 u/gm 1/2 oz tubes	25
*Cephalexin caps 250 mg	200
caps 500 mg	100
*Erythromycin caps 250 mg	1,000
chewable tab 200 mg	1,000
*Griseofulvin tab microsize 200 mg	50
tab microsize 500 mg	50
tab ultramicrosize 125 mg	50
tab ultramicrosize 250 mg	50
*Lotrimin® Solution	40 ml
*Mebendazole tab 100 mg	50
*Monostat-Derm Cream®	50 gm
*Naphcon A® Solution	15 ml
*Neosporin Ophthalmic Ointment 1/8 oz tube	20
Solution 10 ml	20
*Nystatin tab 500,000 u	100
*Oxacillin cap 250 mg	200
cap 500 mg	200
*Penicillin G-benzathine 600,000 u	20
1,200,000 u	20
*Penicillin G-procaine 600,000 u	20
1,200,000 u	20
*Penicillin V tab 250 mg	1,000
tab 500 mg	500
*Sulfacetamide, sodium ophthalmic	
ointment 10% 3.5 gm tube	20
solution 10% 15 ml	20
*Sulfasoxizole tab 500 mg	1,000
*Tetracycline caps 250 mg	1,000
caps 500 mg	500
*Trimethoprim Sulfamethoxazole	
tab 80 mg	200
400 mg	
tab 160 mg	200
800 mg	
*Vasocon A® Solution	15 ml

Anti-Allergic Drugs and Stimulants

*Adrenalin® Epinephrine hydrochloride:	
amp 1:1000 aqueous (30 ml vial)	2
amp 1:200 in suspension (1 ml vial)	5
*Aminophylline: amp 10 ml	2
(Theophylline with ethylenediamine)	
Ammonia inhalant: amp	12

Table I (continued)

*Aramine® amp 1 ml (10 mg/ml)	2
(Metaraminol bitartrate)	
*Hydrocortisone: vials, IV (100 mg/ml for dilution)	3
*Isuprel® (Isoproterenol hydrochloride):	
amp 1:5000 (0.2 mg/ml)	2
*Kenalog 10 (Triamcinolone):	
10 mg/ml. Vial 5 ml	2
*Levophed®, norepinephrine: amp 4 mg/4 ml	2
(Levarterenol bitartrate)	
*Prednisolone: tab 1 mg	20
*Prednisone: tab 5 mg	20

Analgesics, Antipyretics, Sedatives, Antianxiety

Acetaminophen: tab 325 mg	500
Aspirin: tab 300 mg (acetysalicylic acid)	500
Atarax® tab 25 mg	50
*Benztropine mesylate (Cogentin®) tab 1 mg	20
*Codeine: tab 15 mg (codeine sulfate)	25
*Darvon® (dextro-propoxyphene hydrochloride):	
cap 32 mg	25
cap 65 mg	25
*Demerol® (meperidene hydrochloride):	
tab 50 mg	10
amp 50 mg/ml	10
*Diazepam (Valium®) 2 mg	20
5 mg	50
*Haloperidol (Haldol®) 10 ml vial (5 mg/ml)	1 vial
*Imiprimine hydrochloride (Tofranil®) 25 mg	20
*Librium® (chlordiazepoxide)	
tab 25 mg	30
100 mg inject/pack	2 packs
*Lidocaine 1/2% and 1% (20 ml)	2 each
*Morphine sulfate: 20 ml amp (15 mg/ml)	2
*Phenobarbital (Luminol®): tab 15 mg	50
tab 30 mg	20
amp 25 mg	2
*Procyclidine hydrochloride (Kemadrin®)	
tab 2 mg	20
*Seconal® (secobarbital): cap 50 mg	25
amp 50 mg/m	15
Terpin hydrate with codeine	
(cough mixture)	1 pint

Antihistamines

*Alupent® tab 10 mg	50
*Benadryl® (diphenhydramine hydrochloride):	
cap 25 mg	100
vial 10 ml - 50 mg/ml	1
Chlor-Trimeton® (chlorpheniramine maleate)	
tab 4 mg	50
Dimetapp® tab 15 mg	50

Table I (continued)

*Extendryl® cap	50
*Periactin® (cyproheptadine hydrochloride):	
tab 4 mg	100
*PBZ® —PBZ-SR® (tripelennamine	
hydrochloride): tab 50 mg	50
tab 100 mg (delayed action)	50

Ointments

Desenex®	2 lbs
Eucerin®	1 lb
*Hydrocortisone 1%	50 tubes
Ludbriderm®	120 gm
Nupercainal	10 tubes
Polysporin® ointment 1 oz tubes	25 tubes
*Triamcenolone Acetonide Cream:	
0.1% 1/2 oz tube	20 tubes
0.025% 1/2 oz tube	20 tubes
Vaseline (unit dose package)	500
Zinc Oxide - 1 oz tube	50 tubes

Miscellaneous

Alcohol (70%)	1 quart
Airway, oral: adult	1
child	1
*Antivenin package (Black Widow Spider)	2
(Merck, Sharpe & Dohme West Point, PA 19486)	
*Antivenin package (Pit Viper Snakes)	2
(Wyeth Lab., Box 8299, Philadelphia, PA 19101)	
*Auralgan® ear drops - 15 ml bottles	2
Baking Soda	1/2 lb
Betadine Ointment® (unit dose package)	1,000
Betadine Solution® - 8 oz bottles	20
*Calcium gluconate - 10% - vials 10 ml	2
Calomine Lotion	1 pint
*Chloromycetin® otic solution:	
15 ml bottle	1
*Coly-mycin S otic solution - 10 ml bottle	1
*Cortisporin® otic suspension:	
10 ml bottle	5
Debrox® - 30 ml bottle	2
Dramamine® tab 50 mg (dimenhydrinate)	50
*Glucose (5% in saline 500 ml)	2
Hydrogen peroxide	1 pint
*Ipecac, syrup of	120 ml
Milk of Magnesia (30 ml unit dose)	100
Mineral oil (30 ml unit dose)	100
*Otic Demeboro® solution - 60 ml	2
*Saline - normal (sterile) 500 ml	5 bottles
*Sodium bicarbonate - 4.2 g (50 m Eq) per 50 ml vial	2

Table I (continued)

Tincture of Benzoin spray	1 can
solution	1 bottle
*Thorazine® (chlorpromazine) tab 10 mg	20
Tracheostomy tubes adult	1
child	1
*Water - sterile (vials)	10

Surgical Supplies

Ace bandage, 3 inch	10
Adhesive tape, Durapone®	
1/2 in. roll	5
1 in. roll	5
2 in. roll	5
Applicators	500
Band-Aids®	500
Bandage scissors	3
Bard-Parker blades	
No. 11 stab	1 package
No. 12 curved	1 package
curved and stab (mixed)	8
Bard-Parker handle	2
Basin, stainless steel, sterile	2
Cans with covers, stainless steel	3
Cotton sterile	2 lbs
bulk	2 lbs
Coverlet® adhesive dressing:	
2 in. x 1-1/2 in.	25
3 in. x 2-1/2 in.	25
Ear syringe for irrigation	1
Ear syringe (rubber)	1
Finger cots	100
Forceps	8
Forceps, pick-up	1
Gauze, roller 25 ft. x 1 in.	1
10 ft. x 1 in.	5
1(ft. x 2 in.	10
10 ft. x 3 in.	5
Guaze squares 3 in. x 3 in.	500
2 in. x 2 in.	500
Gauze, Vaseline	5
Gloves, rectal	10
Gloves, sterile Size 7	5
Size 7-1/2	5
Size 8	5
Levine tube, plastic	1
Medicine droppers	24
Medicine dropper bottles	24
Needle holder	2
Oval eye pads with shields	6
Pan, small aluminum, sterile for saline or betadine irrigation	3
Scissors	8

Table I (continued)

Splints, padded arms	2
legs	2
Suture 3-0 with needle, nylon	2 packages
4-0 with needle, nylon	2 packages
5-0 with needle PS-2 ethilon nylon	2 packages
5-0 chromic PS-4 needle	2 packages
6-0 chromic PS-4 needle	5 packages
Syringes: TB	10
2 ml	5
5 ml	5
10 ml	5
Tongue depressors	1,000
Towel and drapes, sterile, disposable	5 packages
Wash basin	2

Miscellaneous Equipment

Alcohol preps, Webcol®	1,000
Ambu resuscitator	1
Basin, emesis	2
Bedpans	2
Crutches	2 pr
Hot water bottles	2
Ice bags	1 package
Ipecac, syrup	4 oz
I.V. Sets Medisets and extensions	5
Stopcocks	5
Armboards, several sizes	4
Lamp, infrared	1
Lamp, mobile	1
Magnifying glass	1
Nebulizer	2
Oxygen, small tank	1
Scale	1
Sterilizer	1
Stretcher	1
Thermometer, Tempa Dot®, single use	1,000
Thermometer (oral)	6
Thermometer (rectal)	6
Urinals	2

First aid kits should be supplied to the counselors for overnight camping trips. The following is a suggested list of equipment for a group of about ten campers and three counselors. It is also very important to the Health Supervisor to inform the counselor in charge of the trip about any camper who might be allergic to certain medications and foods, and about any camper who is upon daily medication. The medication for the one- to three-day trip should then be given to the counselor.

TRIPPER'S FIRST AID KIT

	2-3 day Trips	Long Trips 2-3 Weeks
Dressings		
Adhesive 1/2 in. roll	1	10
2 in. roll	1	10
Applicators	15	50
Bandaids®	10	100
Bandages, small	25	50
medium	25	40
Gauze 1 in. roll	2	5
2 in. roll	2	5
Guaze Pads, large	2	10
Steri-Pads, 2 in. x 2 in.	15	30
Medications		
Acetaminophen, 325 mg tablets	10	100
Aspirin, 300 mg tablets	10	100
Betadine®, 30 ml	1	3
Spirits of ammonia	6 vials	12
Miscellaneous		
Bandages scissors, small	1	2
First aid manual	1	1
Razor blade	1	12
Tourniquet	1	2

Chapter IV

COMMON MEDICAL AND SURGICAL PROBLEMS

Fortunately, most medical and surgical problems encountered in camp are not of a serious nature. This can be seen by reviewing *Table II*, which gives the spectrum of problems encountered at the boys' camp where one of the authors served as physician for 12 years. The disorders are listed in two categories—inpatient and outpatient services. As you will note, the number of infirmary admittances is relatively small. As one might guess, the most common medical problems in the outpatient service were upper and lower respiratory infections. Another large category involved bruises, sprains, and abrasions. Other disorders seen with relative frequency were gastroenteritis, asthma, sunburn, and 'athlete's foot.'

The counselor is usually the first person to be faced with the responsibility of making a decision regarding a sick or injured camper. It is not too unusual for a camper to feign illness, especially when faced with a frustrating experience. It is wise for the counselor to take the complaining camper to the nurse, even if it seems that the camper is feigning illness. Sometimes a short visit with an understanding nurse will be curative. The nurse should always be willing to see a camper complaining of illness and to check his temperature. A good nurse will then ask the physician to see the patient if there is any uncertainty in his/her mind about the camper's complaint.

Certain important principles should be stressed regarding the physician's responsibility toward a camper who comes seeking medical help. The physician should certainly be willing to see and, if necessary, examine a camper with a complaint. A camper with fever, regardless of the cause, should be in the infirmary for observation by the nurse and physician, because the illness may be the beginning of a contagious illness, and isolation in the infirmary may be advisable. It is unfair to expect the counselor to shoulder the responsibility and medical care of a sick camper. Although camping life encourages ruggedness, this principle should not apply in time of illness. The parents will have much more peace of mind knowing that their boy or girl with a fever is in the infirmary under the watchful eyes of the Health Supervisor. Finally, the camp infirmary is not truly a hospital. If a camper is sick and the diagnosis is in doubt so that laboratory procedures are in order, it is wise to transfer such a patient to a hospital in a nearby community and seek consultant help.

Before the specific medical and surgical procedures are discussed, a word should be said about drug therapy for the pediatric patient. The Health Supervisor soon becomes aware that the majority of campers come to see the physician with relatively minor complaints, and heroic

Table II

Three-Year Survey

Disease	Number of Patients
Outpatient Service	
1. Upper respiratory infections	405
2. Abrasions, lacerations, bruises	196
3. 'Athlete's foot'	63
4. Headache	60
5. Sprain	53
6. Gastroenteritis	46
7. Asthma	35
8. Sunburn	28
9. Poison Ivy	24
10. Insect bites	24
11. Conjunctivitis	23
12. Acute otitis media	22
13. Blisters	12
14. Foreign body—skin	10
15. Furuncle	9
16. Ingrown toenail	8
17. Laryngitis	8
18. Fever—unknown origin	7
19. Burn	6
20. Plantar wart	5
21. Bronchitis	5
22. Malaise	4
23. Epistaxis	4
24. Fracture	3
25. Toothache	2
26. Eczema	2
27. Paronychia	2
28. Cervical adenitis	2
29. Chipped tooth	1
Inpatient Service	
1. Acute rhinopharyngitis	34
2. Gastroenteritis	9
3. Fever—unknown origin	8
4. Asthma	7
5. Headache—abdominal pain	6
6. Bruise—sprain	5
7. Acute otitis media	4
8. Cuts	4
9. Head injury	2
10. Fatigue	2
11. Fainting	1
12. Poison ivy	1
13. Acute appendicitis	1
14. Infected insect bites	1

measure and enthusiastic drug therapy are not indicated. During the first several weeks of camp, the Health Supervisor will see a number of campers who will come complaining of headache or sore throat or other feigned illness as somatic expressions of homesickness, frustration, or incompatibility with his fellow campers or his counselor. Sympathetic but firm reassurance is good therapy. Also, an occasional placebo or throat lozenge are of inestimable help to the Health Supervisor, counselor, and camper. The camp physician should not attempt to treat a serious illness such as possible meningitis, sepsis, etc., in the camp infirmary. Such a patient should be transferred to a nearby hospital. The Health Supervisor must strive for the maximum factor of safety in treating the campers. The drugs should be given by mouth whenever possible. Parenteral administration is sometimes indicated when the patient is vomiting. The physician must, of course, be acquainted with the therapeutic potential of a drug as well as the possible toxic reactions. He must also be familiar with the dosage and mode of administration of a drug. Most pediatric and adult drug doses can be found in the *Physician's Desk Reference* (PDR) or Appendix II for commonly used medications.

Injuries

Cuts

Any camper who suffers a cut should be taken to the camp Health Supervisor by the counselor. If there is profuse bleeding, the counselor should apply direct pressure with gauze squares from the first aid kit over the bleeding area. If the counselor has no kit available, a clean handkerchief pressed directly upon the cut will suffice until he/she can get the camper to the nurse.

The nurse in turn can offer reassurance to the camper. If there is anxiety or hysteria, aspirin, codeine, or Seconal® may be given to the camper (this should not be given when there is a head injury).

The cut should then be washed thoroughly with soap and water. If the cut does not require sutures, the nurse can apply Betadine® and a bandage. If she is uncertain, or if it is obvious that the cut will need sutures, the physician should see the patient. The nurse should also get the physician's opinion regarding tetanus toxoid or immune globulin administration. When the Health Supervisor sees the camper, he has to make the decision as to whether the camper should be treated at camp or transferred to a hospital. If a cut is extensive or if it involves the face and especially the eyes, or if there is a question of a severed tendon, it is wise to transfer the camper to a hospital and request consultant help.

If a cut is not too extensive and requires three to four sutures, this can be done in the camp infirmary. The wound should be cleansed thoroughly with soap and water and debrided if necessary. Sterile trays (*Table III*) should be kept in the infirmary (it is wise to keep two trays so that one can be on hand while the other is being sterilized).

Table III

Suture Tray (For Small Lacerations)

No. 20 and No. 25 needles	Curved large mosquitos (2)
Needle holder	Curved small mosquitos (2)
Straight suture scissors	Sterile drape
Curved scissors (for debridement)	Gauze flats (8)
	6-0, 4-0, 3-0 nylon suture with saw-edged needle
Mouse-tooth forceps	
Smooth forceps	Syringes, 2 ml and 10 ml
Knife holder	Anesthesia, local (lidocaine, novocaine) 1 ampule
Blades No. 10 and No. 11 (stab)	
	Sterile rubber gloves (sizes 7, 7-1/2, 8)

Prep Tray

Emesis basins (sterile normal saline in one) (2)	Syringe, 2 ml (1)
	Gauze flats (8)
Kelly forceps—large (1)	Betadine® solution

All wounds, especially puncture wounds, should be considered as potentially dangerous, and the possibility of tetanus should be kept in mind. Most camp directors give specific instructions to the parents for the campers to have a booster of tetanus toxoid if indicated before coming to camp, and most campers are adequately immunized. However, if an injury is extensive, dirty, or heavily contaminated, such as an injury sustained in the horseback-riding area, a booster should be given.

(The American Academy of Pediatrics schedule of recommended immunizations is outlined in *Table IV*.) The Health Supervisor must remember that the camp personnel may not have been adequately protected against tetanus. This is especially true of the kitchen help, maintenance staff, and counselors, and they may need passive immunization with human tetanus immune globulin (TIG). The decision as to whether or not to administer tetanus toxoid or tetanus antitoxin should be made by the physician.

Tetanus is a preventable disease, and the effectiveness of prevention is beyond question as a result of the U.S. Armed Forces experience in World War II. Particular attention is directed to No. 5 subtitle of *Table IV* which states that *adult* diphtheria tetanus toxoid should be used for all children over six years of age. This product contains a smaller amount of diphtheria antigen than is present in products used for routine pediatric immunizations of children less than six years of age. The booster

Table IV

Recommended Schedule for Active Immunization of Normal Infants and Children*

Recommended Age	Vaccine(s)	Comments
2 mo	DTP[1], OPV[2]	Can be initiated earlier in areas of high endemicity
4 mo	DTP, OPV	2-mo. interval desired for OPV to avoid interference
6 mo	DTP (OPV)	OPV optional for areas where polio might be imported (e.g., southwest U.S.)
12 mo	Tuberculin Test[3]	May be given simultaneously with MMR at 15 mo.
15 mo	Measles, Mumps, Rubella (MMR)[4]	MMR preferred
18 mo	DTP, OPV	Consider as part of primary series—DPT essential
4-7 yr	DTP, OPV	
14-16 yr	Td[5]	Repeat every 10 years for lifetime

*Report of the Committee on Infectious Diseases—American Academy of Pediatrics, 19th Edition, 1982 (reproduced with permission by the American Academy of Pediatrics).

[1]DTP—Diphtheria and tetanus toxoids with pertussis vaccine.

[2]OPV—Oral, attenuated poliovirus vaccine contains poliovirus types 1, 2, and 3.

[3]Tuberculin Test—Mantoux (intradermal PPD) preferred. Frequency of tests depends on local epidemiology. The Committee recommends annual or biennial testing unless local circumstances dictate less frequent or no testing.

[4]MMR—Live measles, mumps, and rubella viruses in a combined vaccine.

[5]TD—Adult tetanus toxoid (full dose) and diphtheria toxoid (reduced dose) in combination after seventh (7th) birthday.

For all products used, consult manufacturer's brochure for instructions for storage, handling, and administration. Biologics prepared by different manufacturers may vary, and those of the same manufacturer may change from time to time. The package insert should be followed for a specific product.

recommended "tetanus toxoid and time of injury" is predicated on the child having received the initial three diphtheria, tetanus, and pertussis (DTP) and a booster at 18 months of age. If the patient has *not* had the initial three DTP and one DTP booster, a booster of adult tetanus booster (Td) alone may be indicated before the ten years and five years as stated. The administration of tetanus toxoid poses no hazard from the standpoint of allergic reactions.

Tetanus immune globulin (human) (TIG) is a markedly improved product over the equine tetanus antitoxin previously used. It is available commercially, and it is *not* necessary to do sensitivity tests (skin and conjunctival) prior to injection. It is administered intramuscularly and *never* intravenously. Before administering, as with any biological product, the physician should take all precautions known for the prevention of allergic reactions. A review of the patient's history regarding sensitivity and reactions to other biological products should be taken. Epinephrine 1:1000 should be available and ready for use. Local and systemic reactions are infrequent and usually mild. Allergic reactions such as hives and local inflammation may occasionally occur. Shock-like reactions are rare. However, repeated injections of gamma globulin may produce hypersensitivity in allergic individuals. The physician should consider the use of horse serum only if human globulin (TIG) is not available within 24 hours.

The antibiotic of choice in the management of potential Clostridial infection is penicillin G with clindimycin and/or tetracycline as an alternate. A guide to tetanus prophylaxis is summarized in *Table V*. One final word—in the treatment of cuts and abrasions, debridement and cleansing with soap and water is an extremely important part of the overall treatment in the prevention of tetanus and secondary infections.

Removal of Fishhooks

On occasion, fishhooks may become lodged in the skin of a camper. The removal of a fishhook is quite simple. The area should be washed with soap and water and Betadine® applied and infiltrated with procaine. The barbed end of the hook should then be forced through the skin which has been anesthetized. The barbed end of the hook can then be clipped with a wire clipper beyond the curved end of the hook. The shaft of the hook can then be removed with forceps. The tract of the fishhook should then be irrigated with normal saline, and Betadine® solution instilled. The camper should receive an injection of tetanus toxoid, and the Health Supervisor should plan to follow the camper daily until the wound is healed.

Sprains

Sprains are very commonly seen in a summer camp, and treatment is simple in most instances. A sprain is a complete or partial tear or stretch-

Table V

Summary Guide to Tetanus Prophylaxis in Routine Wound Management

History of tetanus immunization (doses)	Clean, minor wounds		All other wounds	
	Td[1]	TIG	Td[1]	TIG
Uncertain	Yes	No	Yes	Yes
0-1	Yes	No	Yes	Yes
2	Yes	No	Yes	No[2]
3 or more	No[3]	No	No[4]	No

[1]For children less than seven years old, DTP (DT, if pertussis vaccine is contraindicated) is preferred to tetanus toxoid alone. For persons seven years old and older, Td (adult diphtheria tetanus toxoid) is preferred to tetanus toxoid alone.

[2]None, if wound is more than 24 hours old.

[3]Yes, if more than ten years since last dose.

[4]Yes, if more than five years since last dose. (More frequent boosters are not needed and can accentuate side effects.)

Tetanus Immune Globulin (Human) (T.I.G.)

  - Prophylaxis - 250 units intramuscularly for children and adults.

Morbidity and Mortality Weekly Report. Center for Disease Control 29:404, August 21, 1981.

---

ing of one or more of the ligaments about a joint and is caused by a sudden twist of the bones which constitute a joint. Pain on movement of the involved joint is the chief complaint. The camper should be taken to the nurse as soon as possible. If this is not possible, immediate application of cold compresses will help reduce the swelling. A well-padded compression bandage should be applied to the injured part and the camper should rest the joint for 24 to 48 hours. After 24 hours, daily heat to the injured area will help. When the camper returns to activity, strapping the affected joint or an ace bandage will help protect it from further injury.

The sequence of events with a sprain are hemorrhage and hematoma formation. The cold application (ice water rather than cracked ice) of compresses help reduce the extent of the swelling. Immobilization will also help reduce the bleeding. When the hematoma is absorbed, there is fibroblastic proliferation. The application of heat will help during the latter phase of the reparative process. During the first 24 hours, it is difficult to do a complete examination of the joint, and is best accomplished after that. In most instances, it is wise to get an opinion from an

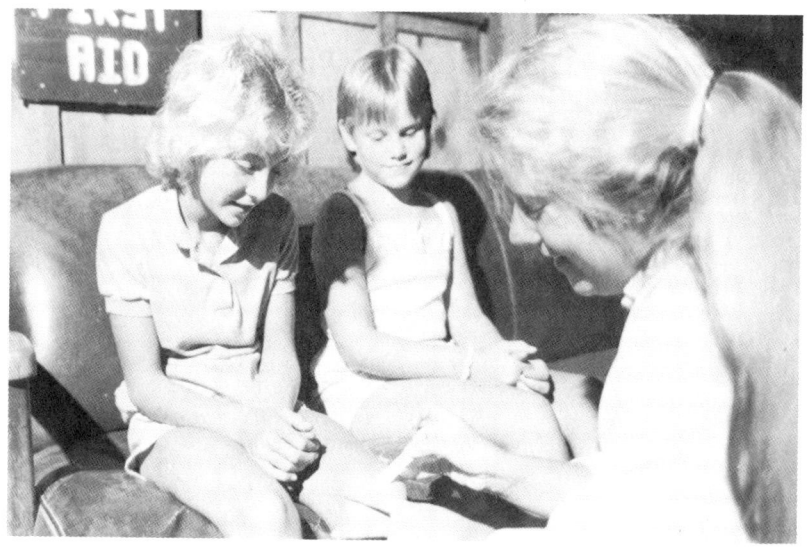

orthopedic surgeon, and roentgenograms should be obtained of the injured area unless the camper shows complete recovery in 24 to 48 hours.

Probably, the most frequent injury is the 'jammed finger.' This injury seems trivial and not incapacitating, but if neglected, it may lead to permanent residual crippling. It is wise to obtain a x-ray to rule out a fracture. The period of immobilization of the injured digit is longer when fractured. With such injuries, it is wise to have the guidance of an orthopedic surgeon.

Strains

A strain is a tear in the muscle, tendon, or fascia. The camper will complain almost immediately of pain. Although the strain may be deep in the muscle, cold applications initially will be helpful. The camper should be taken to the infirmary, where cold applications may be continued for 20 to 30 minutes. Rest to the injured muscle is important, and for the next 24 to 48 hours the application of heat will help. The sequence of events is very similar to sprains. At first there is hemorrhage, and a hematoma forms. There is fibroblastic proliferation during the healing process. If the camper continues to complain after 48 hours, it is wise to get an opinion from an orthopedic surgeon, and x-ray of the injured area should be obtained.

When the camper is injured and there is a high probability of a fractured upper or lower extremity, proper immobilization is important. This type of first aid is well described in a number of first aid manuals. It is wise not to move the patient but to have the nurse come to the scene of the accident. The nurse can check upon the adequacy of the immobilization and extent of the injury and give the patient either aspirin or codeine for pain and discomfort. The physician should make the decision about moving the patient for further diagnostic procedures and treatment.

The treatment of severe injuries and head injuries is taken up in the section on emergencies and need not be covered here.

One general principle should be reemphasized: It is not necessary to get the injured camper to the infirmary immediately. The counselor should make the injured camper as comfortable as possible and get the Health Supervisor to come to the scene, and they will be better able to make the decisions about moving the camper.

Any injury which requires sutures, roentgenograms, or a consultant's opinion should be reported by letter to the parents. The camper usually informs his parents by letter, and the injury is often described in vague or vivid terms. A frantic phone call will follow from the parents unless the Health Supervisor's letter of explanation precedes the camper's note.

Medical Problems

There are a variety of minor medical problems which are commonly encountered at camp. The treatment is simple, and the most important precautionary warning in the management of these relatively mild complaints is not to overlook the possibility of an underlying serious disorder.

Headache

This is a very common complaint, especially during the first several weeks of camp. Many of the young campers will complain of headache when in reality they are homesick or are incompatible with their peers or their counselor. The counselor should make certain that the camper who complains of a headache has not been injured. The camper may be fatigued, and the counselor should have the camper rest for 30 to 60 minutes. If the complaint persists, or if there are associated complaints or symptoms, such as sore throat, cough, fever, etc., the camper should be taken to see the nurse. The nurse should examine the camper's head for evidence of trauma and check the camper's temperature. If the headache is feigned, the trip to the infirmary and a little visit with a firm but sympathetic nurse will often cure the camper. If the camper is febrile and has other complaints such as a sore throat, the headache is usually part of the symptom complex of infection, and the camper should be examined by the physician.

Abdominal Pain

This too is a very common complaint, especially in campers who are homesick, frustrated, or who have had squabbles with their peers or counselor. If the complaint of abdominal pain is not accompanied by fever, nausea, vomiting, or diarrhea, the camper can be handled by an understanding counselor. If the complaint persists or is associated with other signs or symptoms, the camper should be taken to the infirmary.

The camper should be seen by the nurse and his temperature should be checked. If the abdominal pain is feigned, the nurse can usually take care of the camper. It must be stressed that a complaint of abdominal pain should never be ignored. The complaint may be a manifestation of pharyngitis, tonsillitis, bronchitis, or gastroenteritis, and on rare occasions may be due to acute appendicitis. A good nurse should be able to decide when a camper should be examined by the physician. If the patient is febrile, he should rest in the infirmary where he can be examined and followed by the physician and nurse. A period of observation and examination by the physician will usually solve the problem. If the physician feels that the abdominal pain is due to acute pharyngitis, tonsillitis, or gastroenteritis, appropriate medication can be started. If the abdominal pain persists and is associated with slight fever, vomiting, and especially if there is localization of the pain in the right lower abdominal quadrant, do not give the camper a laxative or aspirin. It is best to transfer the patient to a hospital as a case of possible appendicitis.

The above advice should apply to the counselor who is on a trip when a camper develops persistent abdominal pain. The thought of appendicitis can be especially frightening to the counselor who is isolated in the woods on a trip. It might be reassuring to the counselor that appendicitis is rarely encountered in a camp setting. For example, only one camper with appendicitis was seen in 12 years by one of us.

Vomiting

Vomiting as an isolated sign usually is not difficult to handle. An occasional camper may overeat or vomit from overexertion. A half-hour of rest will usually take care of the difficulty. If vomiting persists, the counselor should take the camper to the infirmary. The Health Supervisor should have the camper rest. His temperature should be checked. Initially, it is best to give him nothing by mouth. This could be followed by ice chips and then small amounts of cold water or a carbonated beverage. Vomiting may be a manifestation of an acute pharyngitis or tonsillitis, and if the camper is febrile, he should be examined by the physician. If the vomiting is a manifestation of gastroenteritis, diarrhea will follow. The Health Supervisor should then look for other campers who might have eaten contaminated food. Generalized abdominal pain will usually accompany vomiting, and the possibility of an acute appendicitis should be kept in mind by the Health Supervisor. Careful observation in the infirmary and frequent examinations will help establish this diagnostic possibility.

Diarrhea

This complaint in an isolated camper is not serious, but the camper should be admitted to the infirmary.

If a camper complains of diarrhea, it is wise to cut down on his food intake. The diarrhea is usually self-limiting and will subside within 24 hours. In most instances, the cause cannot be found, and diet restriction will control the diarrhea. If the diarrhea is unusually severe, it may be wise to admit the camper to the infirmary for one to two days. State health laboratories will accept stool cultures, and this service should be used, especially if the diarrhea persists beyond two days.

Food Poisoning

An episode of vomiting and diarrhea is always worrisome to the Health Supervisor because of its implications as a potential threat to the health and safety of the entire camp. The conscientious Health Supervisor quickly thinks about the water supply, sewage disposal, health of the kitchen staff, and possible contaminated food as a source. Fortunately, in most well-run camps this rarely poses a serious threat and food poisoning is rarely a source of serious difficulty. Gastroenteritis, however, is encountered at camp, and it is well for the physician to have a clear understanding about the term *food poisoning*.

The term *food poisoning* is applied to the condition characterized chiefly by acute gastroenteritis which develops within a few hours after ingestion of food or drink which contains one of the following materials:

1. Living microorganisms which release toxins and which multiply in the intestine (infectious type of food poisoning);
2. Toxins which have been formed by bacteria before ingestion—no living organism present (toxic food poisoning);
3. Poisonous chemicals such as salts of arsenic, lead, and zinc, or toxic animals or plants such as mushrooms, poisonous fish, or mussels that have subsisted on alkaloid-containing plankton.

If an explosive outbreak of vomiting and diarrhea occurs at a camp, so that one-third to one-half of the camp residents are affected, the following operating procedure is practical and effective. Most infirmaries are inadequate to care for all those affected. It is best to have the campers and counselors remain in their cabins, and the Health Supervisor can make the rounds and care for all those affected. It is best to provide each cabin with No. 10 cans which can serve as containers for vomitus. Those with diarrhea will have to use the toilet facilities. It is also a good idea to provide each cabin with liquid soap, a mop, and water to clean up any vomitus upon the floor. Restriction of food is indicated—chipped ice is beneficial. Sedatives such as Seconal® for those who are apprehensive are helpful. Any patient who may become dehydrated should be admitted to the infirmary.

The following additional steps should be taken:

1. It is usually difficult to find an obvious cause, but the water, sewage disposal, and milk supply should be checked to see if any break in sanitation has occurred. It is wise to call in the district health officer as a consultant in such a situation.
2. All kitchen personnel should be examined for evidence of pyogenic skin infections, and throat cultures should be sent to the state laboratory.
3. The Health Supervisor should make a statement of reassurance to the campers and personnel that the problem is not serious and can be controlled. This is extremely important for morale purposes.

Although typhoid, paratyphoid, or bacillary dysentery will seldom be the cause of explosive episodes of diarrhea in a camp, the physician should think of these infections as possibilities. It is for this reason that short summaries describing these infections are included in Appendix I.

Rectal Bleeding

This is most often due to either hemorrhoids or an anal fissure, and it is wise to have the camper examined by a physician. If this is due to a fissure and/or hemorrhoids, an anesthetic ointment such as Nupercainal® will give symptomatic relief. Encouraging the camper to increase his water and vegetable intake will help prevent constipation. If the bleeding persists; it is wise to get the help of a consultant.

Blood in Urine

This is potentially serious, especially if it persists for more than one day, and the camper should either be sent home or to a hospital where a thorough evaluation can be carried out.

Fever

Fever is almost always a manifestation of infection, and the camper will usually have complaints such as headache, sore throat, etc. Any camper with fever should be admitted to the infirmary for observation, diagnosis, and treatment. The fever may be treated with aspirin or symptomatic relief until a diagnosis is made and then specific medication prescribed.

Toothache

Toothache is usually caused by injury, i.e., chipped tooth, and all that is indicated is administration of an analgesic drug such as aspirin or acetaminophen. If the camper has rampant caries, an apical root abscess might be the cause of the toothache, and again aspirin or acetominophen will afford symptomatic relief. Dental consultation should be obtained, and antibiotic therapy may be indicated.

Motion Sickness

This is preventable in most instances. Upon the camp physical examination blanks there should be a notation regarding the camper's susceptibility to motion sickness, and a list of names of these campers should be posted in the infirmary. Prior to automobile trips, the Health Supervisor should give the campers the appropriate dose of Dramamine® (see Appendix II for dose).

Fainting

Fainting may have a variety of causes, such as severe emotional stress, excitement, the sight of blood, or from being forced to stand too long in one place. Upon occasion, this will accompany micturition. The treatment is simple: allow the camper to remain flat on his back. Wash his face with cool water. A whiff of aromatic spirits of ammonia will help. Consciousness will return promptly. If consciousness does not return promptly, or if fainting tends to recur, the cause may be serious. In either case, the camper should have a thorough physical examination, including a neurologic examination. An isolated episode of fainting needs no more discussion, but if the fainting tends to recur or if there are abnormal neurologic findings, the camper should be seen by a neurologist in consultation and probably sent home for further evaluation.

Pediculosis (Body Lice)

This is an infestation with adult lice, larvae, or nits of the scalp and hairy parts of the body and is caused by Pediculus humanus, head louse or body louse, and Phthirus pubis, crab louse. The infestation is transmitted by direct contact with an infected person or indirectly with clothing from an infested person. The eggs hatch in a week and reach maturity in two weeks isolation of the camper is not necessary. Treatment is usually effective if the regimen in Appendix I, page 136 is followed.

Constipation

Constipation might be more correctly classified as a complaint rather than as a disease except in relatively rare conditions. We would strongly discourage the treatment of constipation with laxatives or enemas. We would rather suggest that intake of liquids be increased if a camper comes into the infirmary with this kind of complaint. In the twelve years when one of us served as a camp physician, not a single camper had to be treated for constipation. However, if a camper arrives at camp with instructions to use Metamucil for constipation, it would be advisable for the nurse or camp physician to follow these instructions.

Chapter V

PSYCHIATRIC DISORDERS

by Barbara Herjanic, M.D.
Associate Professor of Child Psychiatry
Washington University School of Medicine

Introduction

The expected incidence of behavioral or emotional disorders in a camp setting is low. Of a total population of 500 campers, including staff, probably fewer than five individuals would have a psychiatric disturbance of such severity that medical intervention would be required. The more serious disorders tend to interfere so much with adjustment in a regular camp setting that children who are seriously disturbed would very likely attend a special camp or stay at home.

However, there are some children with mild to moderately severe disorders of various kinds who will be sent to a regular camp. Sometimes parents look upon camp as a way of improving their child's behavior or giving themselves a needed rest. It is important that a camp physician have sufficient knowledge about psychiatric conditions to be able to handle these wisely should the need arise. It is also important to keep in mind that each individual who comes to camp brings with him a well developed personality and way of behaving, which one cannot expect to change very much during the temporary exposure to camp life.

Many mild behavior problems are handled effectively by counselors and other camp staff and probably never come to the attention of the physician. Medical intervention may only be required when the child's behavioral or emotional disturbance is sufficiently severe and lasting to interfere with his relationships with peers and adults at camp and with his participation in the camp program. Unusually impulsive or bizarre behavior which may endanger the child or those around him requires prompt intervention. The doctor's opinion will be of primary importance in determining whether a disturbed child may stay at camp, should be hospitalized, or should be sent home.

Anxiety Disorders

These disorders are manifested by excessive amounts of anxiety which interfere with the child's functioning. Anxiety is shown by crying, clinging, screaming, or refusal to move, speak, or participate in interaction with others in an appropriate manner. Sometimes physical symptoms such as headache, nausea, vomiting, and abdominal pains are manifestations of anxiety. Young children sometimes show anxiety by temper displays. In older adolescents and young adults, anxiety may be manifested by such symptoms as palpitation, sweating, rapid pulse, dilated pupils, tingling of the extremities, tightness or pain in the chest, and choking or smothering sensations.

A. Homesickness (Separation Anxiety Disorder)

Children with a severe form of this disorder will be unlikely ever to get to camp because they refuse to leave home. However, milder forms may not appear until the child is actually away from home. He then becomes very unhappy, with crying, physical complaints, and repeated and anxious demands to be taken back home immediately.

Treatment of this condition can usually be handled by an understanding counselor, who will try to involve the child in camp activities to take his mind off thoughts of home. Occasionally, it is necessary to reassure a child by allowing him to call home. If this happens and parents support the idea that the child should return home immediately, the camp personnel have little choice in the matter. If parents are supportive of the camp's efforts to help the child work through this uncomfortable situation, then they will refuse to have the child return home. The efforts of the counselor to involve the child in camp life will usually be effective, and the symptoms will gradually disappear. Nighttime may be particularly difficult for these children, and in some instances medication may be useful for a few nights to enable the child to get to sleep.

Symptomatic relief of separation anxiety may be attained by the administration of 25 to 75 mg of imipramine (Tofranil®), starting with 25 mg at bedtime, and increasing gradually until symptoms are relieved. Maximum daily dose should not exceed 5 mg/kg of body weight. Once the child participates actively in the camp program, the drug can be slowly withdrawn.

B. Avoidant Disorder

The child with this disorder shows persistent and excessive shrinking from contact with strangers and may cling to one person in the camp, usually an adult, and refuse to be involved with others. This child has a desire for affection and acceptance, but is too anxious to mingle with a group. This condition would rarely interfere with social functioning to a severe degree in a child who comes to camp. However, any child who is excessively clinging to one person at camp needs an unusual amount of help in learning to interact with a variety of people, particularly with peers.

Treatment consists of an understanding but neutral approach, with care taken not to reinforce the clinging behavior. Efforts should be made to help the child to relate first to another child on an individual basis, and later to participate in group activities.

C. Overanxious Disorder

Children with this disorder are troubled with excessive worries. They may worry about each camp activity before taking part in it, or about past events or past behaviors of their own. They show an excessive concern about their abilities and need a lot of reassurance. They are very likely to have somatic complaints, such as headaches or stomachaches, for which no physical basis can be established. They tend to be markedly self-conscious and susceptible to easy embarrassment or humiliation. They may experience marked feelings of tension or inability to relax. The child usually has had this condition for months prior to the camp experience, but the new setting may precipitate an exacerbation. Most children with this disorder will improve as they become accustomed to camp life.

There is no specific treatment for this disorder, except to recognize that the child needs a great deal of reassurance, and sometimes may have to be individually led or pushed into participation in activities about which he or she feels very anxious.

D. Panic Disorder

The manifestations of this disorder are panic attacks which recur frequently on very slight provocation or for no apparent reason. The symptoms include dyspnea, palpitations, chest pain, choking sensations, dizziness, feelings of unreality, tingling in the hands and feet, hot or cold flashes, sweating, faintness, trembling, and fear of dying or of losing one's mind. The attack may be precipitated by some predetermined stimulus, such as the thought of seeing blood, a fire, or a dead animal. This disorder is usually not found in children, but appears in late adolescence and early adult life. It may cause the subject to avoid situations which he or she has learned previously will bring on the panic symptoms.

Treatment during camp is symptomatic. Usually the precipitant can be avoided or the symptoms can be relieved temporarily by the administration of diazepam (Valium®) in doses of 5 to 10 mg once or twice a day. The person with panic attacks should be encouraged to have a full evaluation and treatment upon return home.

E. Phobias

Children often have specific phobias such as undue fear of spiders, snakes, water, going into the woods, or riding in a boat. Socially related phobias such as fear of crowds, marked fear of being alone, or fears of performing in public tend to affect adolescents and older individuals. Phobias are usually marked by anticipatory anxiety and will often prevent a person from participating in an activity in which he expects to meet up with the feared object or situation. Exposure to a phobic stimulus may precipitate a panic attack.

Unless the phobia interferes seriously with the child's functioning at camp, it probably should be ignored. In a group setting, other children will often help a child to overcome a specific fear. If the phobia interferes with participation in camp activities, desensitization can be done by very gradual introduction of the child to the feared object or situation. Children with phobias do not usually respond to punishment or threats. Understanding, patience, and persistence are required by the camp counselor who is going to help the child face the feared situation. Medication is not advised, unless panic attacks occur in response to the phobic stimulus.

Behavior Disorders

Children bring to camp their individual temperaments and personalities, their learned behaviors, their expectations of adult responses to them, and all of the results of a wide variety of parental guidance and teaching skills. In a large group of children it is sometimes difficult to distinguish those with serious behavioral problems which may indicate a specific disorder from the children who are manifesting the kinds of behavior which may be accepted at home or in other situations but which create difficulties in a camp.

A child who truly has a disorder of behavior needs special attention and may require medication. If a child with a behavior disorder comes to camp with prescribed medications, these should be administered regularly to help this child make as good an adjustment as possible. It is not wise for the camp physician to discontinue a previously prescribed medication even though he may think that the child does not need it. A carefully written report to the parents on the child's behavior and adjustment at camp may be of great value to the family doctor in making decisions about changing the previous treatment when the child returns home.

A. Attention Deficit Disorder with Hyperactivity ('The Hyperactive Child')

Attention deficit disorder is manifested by a marked degree of inattentiveness, impulsivity, and hyperactivity. The child who is only inattentive or impulsive may get along reasonably well at camp, but those with hyperactivity in addition are likely to run into difficulties in peer relationships, in following instructions, in being compliant with the camp rules, and in organizing their activities sufficiently to benefit from the camp program. The child with attention deficit disorder is one who does not catch on readily to instructions given to the group. He tends to be noncompliant, he may run off from the boundaries set for the group, may shift activity quickly, and may talk out and interrupt frequently. He may be the one who climbs trees, races ahead up the hill toward the cliff, and has difficulty recognizing what is dangerous as opposed to what is safe. This condition may be aggravated by the excitement in the camp program. The child may greatly overreact when some new activity is proposed, but he may not stick with one activity long enough to learn a new skill. The hyperactive children are usually not very popular with their peers because they tend to interfere with the normal progression of planned activities.

If the child comes to camp with prescribed medications, this should be administered by the nurse or physician on a regular basis. The most commonly used medication, methylphenidate (Ritalin®), is short-acting and will wear off in three and a half to four hours. Therefore, skipping a dose will cause a deterioration in the child's behavior and performance. Initiation of the drug therapy at camp would be inappropriate.

Hyperactive children often respond to a behavior modification approach if a member of the camp staff has had training in this specialized technique. This requires individualized supervision and direction and should always be on a positive plane.

The hyperactive child needs a great deal of supervision to keep him from impulsively doing something which might be dangerous to himself or to others. The goal in management should be his protection and optimum participation in camp activities during his stay. There is little likelihood that the disorder will be affected in any perceptible way by his being at camp. It probably is wise to place emphasis on socialization and helping the child to get along with his peers. A hyperactive child who is not controlled by any of the above measures should be sent home with advice to his parents to seek professional help.

B. Conduct Disorder

Children with conduct disorder are those who tend to upset other individuals in their environment, but who experience little, if any, inner discomfort or pain related to their behavior or its outcome. A child with conduct disorder tends to repeat antisocial acts over and over again and shows little response to punishment.

The nonaggressive child with a conduct disorder has problems in following rules; he tends to run away, to lie, to steal, to blame others for his difficulties, and he feels very little guilt or remorse. The more aggressive children will attack others. They become known very quickly as the ones who start fights. They fight to win and may injure another child. They are destructive of their own and other people's property.

1. *Stealing* is a symptom of conduct disorder which may cause considerable consternation in the camp setting, and it is a very difficult pattern of behavior to correct. In contrast to emotional disorders, which should be handled privately between the counselor or camp doctor and the child, stealing is something that can best be handled with a group approach. Lecturing the child or telling him that it is wrong, or trying to get him to admit his guilt, will be of no avail. When the stolen goods are found in the possession of a child, that should be enough evidence to call for a meeting of the tent or cottage mates, and bring the problem out into the open for group discussion. Sometimes children with a conduct disorder

will respond better to group and peer pressure than they will to punishment or admonition on the part of an adult. If group pressure proves to be of no avail and the child continues to steal, he should be sent home.

2. *Fire setting* is another behavior which, of course, cannot be tolerated. Usually children who enjoy setting fires can obtain an outlet for this through normal camp activities such as helping to build a bonfire or learning how to start a fire without matches. However, a child who is found to be lighting matches surreptitiously or who has set even one fire in an inappropriate way must be sent home for the safety of the camp. Fire setting is not a behavior that can be corrected easily and requires more than the camp experience and peer pressure to bring it under control.

3. *Sexual "acting out" behavior*—Occasionally an aggressive child with conduct disorder will try to involve other children in sexual play or overt heterosexual or homosexual activity. This can be handled through group meetings, bringing the activity out into the open, discussing it freely, and involving peer pressure to keep the activity at a minimum. Since sexual activity is usually carried out in secret, there probably is a certain amount of this that goes on without the knowledge of the counselors, particularly in camps for teenagers. The Health Supervisor may have opportunities to be involved in discussions of sexual behavior and to answer questions about the physical, social, and emotional aspects of sex. It would be wise for the Health Supervisor, particularly in an adolescent camp, to prepare himself ahead of time by reading some of the many books available on sex education for adolescents, and to practice discussing these topics prior to attending camp.

Serious sexual acting out, such as rape or assault, would be an indication for dismissing the youngster from camp. The camp authorities should notify the police because of the legal implications of such behavior.

Other Disorders

A. Sleep Disorders

1. *Sleepwalking*—This condition usually begins at about the age of four, and recurs at irregular intervals. It affects boys more frequently than girls. It should be noted on the pre-camp medical report so that sleepwalkers are identified when they come to camp. The sleepwalking usually occurs within the first three hours of sleep. The child has a blank staring face, is relatively unresponsive to the efforts of others to communicate with him, and can be awakened only with great difficulty. Upon awakening, the individual may remember parts of a dream but does not know where he went or what he did. There is no impairment of mental activity or behavior following awakening from the sleepwalking episode. Before being awakened there is danger that the sleepwalker may be injured by falling, stumbling, or running into something.

The treatment consists of awakening the sleepwalker, if possible, and keeping a close watch on him so that he does not get injured. The sleepwalker is likely to be back in bed asleep within a half hour of the onset of the episode.

2. *Sleep terror*—This condition is manifested by repeated episodes of abrupt awakening lasting one to ten minutes and usually occurs within the first three hours of onset of sleep. The sleep terror begins with a panicky scream and the individual shows evidence of intense anxiety with increased heart rate, rapid breathing, dilated pupils, sweating, and sometimes piloerection. Children with sleep terrors are unresponsive to efforts of others to comfort or reassure them, and they tend to be confused and disoriented. They may show perseverative movements, such as picking at the pillow. The disorder is probably more frightening to people watching it than to the individual concerned, because the child does not remember the episode afterwards.

Some children respond well to the administration of imipramine (Tofranil®) from 25 to 50 mg at bedtime. This can be tried with parental permission. If the diagnosis cannot be made with certainty and the possibility of night seizures is suspected, then the child should be referred for neurological consultation.

B. Eating Disorders

1. *Anorexia nervosa* is probably the most serious adolescent eating disorder. It is much more likely to be found in girls than boys and it should be recognized early so that the child can receive adequate treatment before becoming seriously ill. The main manifestations are an intense fear of becoming obese which is undiminished by weight loss; a disturbance of body image, shown by the claim of feeling fat even when emaciated; and finally, a weight loss of at least 25 percent of the original body weight. Anorectic girls refuse to maintain body weight over a minimum normal weight for age and height. No physical illness can account for the weight loss. With post-pubertal girls there is usually a cessation of menses.

Anorexia nervosa is an illness in which both physical and psychological factors are combined in a very serious and potentially fatal condition. Because of the psychological factors, an anorectic girl may eat more normally at camp away from her family than she does at home. It is necessary to differentiate between an anorectic, who fears becoming obese, and a depressed adolescent whose main concerns have to do with self-reproach, suicidal ideas, and wishing to die. However, there is sometimes a mixture of depression with features of anorexia.

A very thin individual who is weight-conscious and who limits food intake may be able to make an adequate adjustment at camp. However, such a person should be weighed at least once a week to make sure that the weight is being maintained adequately. Any change in the person's eating habits, such as eating less or food refusal, warrants prompt medical intervention. As the condition is usually longstanding and continues indefinitely, evidence of loss of weight during camp is an indication for returning the child home for intensive treatment.

2. *Bulimia*—This condition also is more common in girls than boys, and is believed to be a variant of anorexia nervosa. These persons are usually weight conscious and wish to lose weight, but they have a pattern of recurrent episodes of binge eating, i.e., eating excessive amounts of food in a short period of time. Following a binge they often feel depressed and self-deprecating, and will make themselves vomit or will take laxatives to rid their bodies of the excess food. The binge eater may experience abdominal pain, sleep interruption, and a great amount of discomfort relating to feeling too full and being bloated. There are frequently wide weight fluctuations.

This is a chronic condition and cannot be definitively managed in a camp. It is not likely to be discovered, as there is a tendency for the binge eater to hide the activity. However, should a youngster come to the attention of the camp physician because of abdominal pain, sleep disturbance, or vomiting, a careful history of eating habits may reveal the bulimia and the necessity for psychiatric intervention. The fact that the binge eating has been brought out into the open may be sufficient to control it during the camp period. However, this individual's weight gain or loss during camp would be an indication for return home for treatment.

3. *Pica*—This is the persistent eating of inedible objects, and is more typical of the preschool child. It would, therefore, be an unusual condition in a camp. However, there are older children, usually from deprived backgrounds or with mental retardation, who will put unusual objects into their mouths and eat them.

Treatment includes prohibition from eating inedible materials. A positive behavioral approach with rewards for not picking up or eating nonnutritive substances may be helpful. However, an absolute end to the problem probably cannot be attained at camp. The condition should be called to the attention of the parents on return home so that further treatment can be instituted.

C. Enuresis

Many enuretic children will avoid going to camp. Other children with enuresis have been able to control the condition for the duration of camp. There is little that can be done effectively to treat the condition at camp, but care should be taken to avoid embarrassment and humiliation of the child in the presence of his peers. Special arrangements for taking care of wet clothing and sheets should be made in as inconspicuous a manner as possible. Some children are helped greatly by the administration of imipramine (Tofranil®) 25 to 50 mg at bedtime. This medication can be used with the parents' permission for the duration of camp. Tofranil® does not cure enuresis, but it often relieves the condition symptomatically and is relatively safe if given in doses no larger than 50 mg per day.

D. Encopresis

Soiling is another condition which is very likely to prevent a child from having a camp experience. However, some children who have recovered from encopresis may have an occasional soiling "accident" while at camp, due to unusual excitement and change in scheduling of their daily habits. If the child has been treated for encopresis before entering camp, information should be obtained from the parents about success in controlling the problem. It is particularly important to know if the child retains stool and needs a laxative. If a scheduled time for bowel movements has been a part of the treatment regime, this should be adhered to at camp.

Encopresis is not a condition which can be cured at camp and soiling should be treated as an "accident." A shower and clean clothes should be provided and the least possible attention drawn to the child because of the condition. Some encopretic children, usually boys, will soil their pants, and appear to be completely oblivious to the smell and the mess. Should a counselor at camp notice the typical smell of the child who has soiled, he/she should take him to the camp cottage and see that he is cleaned up appropriately before returning to the group. The child should not be subject to public attention, humiliation, or made to feel badly because of a problem over which he actually has no voluntary control.

Affective Disorders, Suicidal Behavior, and Psychosis

A. Depression

Preadolescent children rarely have the cluster of signs and symptoms of an actual depressive illness. However, they often respond to disturbing situations in life with various degrees of unhappiness, manifested by a variety of symptoms, such as increased irritability, crying, temporary withdrawal, refusal to participate, refusal to talk, and sometimes threats to do bodily harm to themselves or someone else. In an unhappy child these symptoms tend to be temporary and quickly forgotten, as the situation which brought about the unhappiness changes.

Depressive illness is unlikely to occur in the camp setting, where the children and adolescents experience relief from whatever tensions they live under at home and school, and where most of the activities are geared toward enjoyment and entertainment. However, it is very important for the Health Supervisor to be able to recognize depression. Symptoms include a dysphoric mood or loss of interest or pleasure in almost all usual activities and pastimes, either a decreased appetite with weight loss or a markedly increased appetite with significant weight gain, slowing down of motor activity and thoughts, or agitation and an inner feeling of restlessness. Other symptoms include a change in sleep pattern, involving marked difficulty falling asleep or a tendency to wake up during the night or early in the morning and not be able to go back to sleep. There may be loss of energy and increased fatigue. The depressed person often expresses feelings of worthlessness, self-reproach, and excessive or inappropriate guilt. There may be a change in the person's ability to concentrate or to make decisions. Often a depressed person has recurrent thoughts of death, wishes to be dead, or feels that other people would be better off without him. Such preoccupations may lead to a suicide attempt.

When there are signs or symptoms of depression, the physician must always inquire about suicidal thoughts. All expressions of suicidal thought, intent, and all suicidal acts, no matter how trivial they appear to be, must be taken seriously, even if the person gives an apparently plausible explanation for the depressed state.

If the presenting complaint is a suicidal act, one must inquire about signs and symptoms of depression, as well as the intent behind the act. Signs of hopelessness, a poor outlook toward the future, self-deprecation, and a history of suicide in the family are all important in assessing suicidal risk.

Treatment of depression depends upon a very careful history. If an individual is not suicidal and has responded well to an antidepressant medication in the past, this can be prescribed and probably will give relief, enabling the person to stay at camp. Antidepressant medications are not indicated for emergency treatment, and should not be administered for the first time without consultation with a psychiatrist. A persistent depressive episode in a person with no previous history of depression is an indication for psychiatric referral.

Suicide attempts at camp must be taken very seriously, and any attempt is an indication for returning the child home, with advise to the parents to seek psychiatric treatment. Some children appear to be scratching their wrists, or tying a rope around their necks, or showing unduly dangerous types of behavior for purposes of attracting attention. However, any such behavior is an indication for psychiatric consultation and probably dismissal from camp. There are many opportunities for a child to harm himself in a camp setting if the desire is there.

B. Mania

Although a manic episode is extremely unlikely to occur at camp, the physician should be well enough acquainted with the symptoms to have a high index of suspicion. A manic disorder is manifested by a distinct period of predominantly elevated, expansive, or irritable mood. The behavior shown during a manic episode involves increase in activity with physical restlessness, unusual talkativeness and pressure to keep talking, flight of ideas or the feeling that one's thoughts are racing, and a decreased need for sleep. The manic individual is highly distractible and will often manifest behaviors which have a high potential for painful consequences, such as going on buying sprees, acting out sexually, driving recklessly, or showing otherwise uncharacteristic behaviors. The manic individual may become obsessed with delusions of grandeur or hallucinations relative to his manic thinking and show very bizarre behavior in response to the delusions.

An individual with mania needs immediate medical attention and this should be carried out in a psychiatric hospital, where appropriate tests can be done and where the person can be protected from his bizarre and unusual behaviors. Emergency treatment of a manic patient prior to hospitalization consists of one-to-one supervision in a quiet place where the patient can be protected. Haloperidol (Haldol®), starting with 10 to 30 mg IM, up to a 60 mg total daily dosage, can be given. To prevent extrapyramidal reactions, concomitant administration of oral procyclidine (Kemadrin®) in doses of 2 to 2.5 mg three times a day or 1 to 2 mg of benztropine mesylate (Cogentin®) two to three times a day should be given.

C. Acute Psychosis

The word "psychosis" indicates a condition in which there is gross impairment in reality testing; that is, the individual incorrectly evaluates the accuracy of his or her perceptions and thoughts and makes incorrect inferences about external reality, even in the face of contrary evidence. Delusions and hallucinations without insight into their pathological nature are present. Speech may be incoherent, and the person may be agitated and inattentive. In organic psychosis, disorientation, loss of recent memory, and a fluctuating state of consciousness are present. In nonorganic (functional) psychosis, orientation and memory are usually intact. A psychotic break is usually unmistakable because of the bizarreness of symptoms. The person is unable to respond in a sensible fashion to questions, unable to take part in activities, and unamenable to reasoning or normal forms of communication.

If the camper or staff member is found to be behaving in such a bizarre fashion that he is obviously out of touch with reality, immediate steps need to be taken to have the person removed to a safe place where he can be adequately treated. If the behavior is not too agitated or threatening, it is possible to treat such a person with tranquilizers in the camp infirmary until parents can come to take him home. If the behavior is of a threatening nature, hospitalization in the nearest psychiatric facility should be arranged as quickly as possible.

Rapid relief of disturbing symptoms can be attained by intramuscular injection of 5 to 10 mg of haloperidol (Haldol®) hourly, up to a total of 60 mg, if needed, during the first 24 hours. To prevent dystonic reaction, Cogentin® or Kemadrin® can be administered as described under Mania. A careful record of the indications for emergency treatment, the medicattons, restraints, and other procedures must be kept for medico-legal purposes.

Substance Abuse: Intoxication and Withdrawal Symptoms

Patterns of substance abuse change continually. During the 1960s and early 1970s there was a marked increase in substance abuse. Girls caught up with boys in some forms of abuse. As drugs became popular, the abuse spread to younger age levels and even into elementary schools. In the mid 1970s there was a leveling off of the use of lysergic acid diethylamide (LSD). At the same time there was an increase in use of alcohol, marijuana, phencyclidine (PCP), and cocaine. The National Institute on Drug Abuse reported in 1977 that 53 percent of youths, ages 12 through 17, had had some experience with alcohol, and 28 percent had used marijuana. Usage rates climb with age from the middle teens through the mid-twenties. Statistically, a camp staff member is more likely than a camper to be involved in substance abuse. Drug education programs in the schools may be stemming the tide to some extent, especially among the very young.

The Health Supervisor may be called upon to participate in drug education programs. Information about behavioral and legal matters and long-term effects of abuse can be found in the reference materials. This chapter will cover only medical emergencies relating to substance abuse.

It is important to remember that states of intoxication, delirium, acute psychosis, or coma can be caused by one of several drugs or a combination. One usually cannot be sure which drugs have been taken or in what amounts. Initial treatment has to be aimed at symptom relief and protection of the affected individuals from self-destruction or assaultive behavior. Unless the symptoms are mild, the history clear as verified by witnesses, and one-to-one observation can be provided in the camp, the safest procedure is to administer emergency treatment and transport the patient to the nearest hospital or drug treatment facility.

Emergency measures for the comatose patient include airway maintenance, monitoring vital signs, and starting intravenous fluids. If the patient is conscious, gastric lavage should be done, or emesis provoked by 15 ml of syrup of ipecac orally. If the patient is assaultive, physical restraint should be used. All procedures must be carefully recorded.

Specimens of blood (10 ml.), urine (100 ml.), and stomach contents, if available, should be saved and sent with the patient to the hospital.

A. *Alcohol*—Alcohol use in a camp setting is more likely to cause problems in behavioral management and discipline, rather than medical problems. However, three conditions related to alcohol might come to the physician's attention: (a) acute intoxication, (b) serious overdose, and (c) alcohol withdrawal delirium (D.T.'s).

Acute intoxication is a familiar condition in which the odor of alcohol on the breath and/or a history of recent drinking confirms the diagnosis.

This condition is best handled by placement in a quiet room with continuous supervision and adequate fluids until the intoxication subsides.

Overdose of alcohol can be dangerous in a child or young person due to central nervous system depression. Alcohol and drugs may have been ingested together. Attention has to be given to cardiorespiratory functioning. If a young person is in a non-arousable state for any reason, life support measures must be instituted and hospitalization arranged.

Alcohol withdrawal delirium is a serious condition and has been reported in children. A long history of alcoholism is not a prerequisite. D.T.'s usually occur two to three days after cessation of drinking; therefore, it is most likely to occur soon after arrival at camp. The patient should be given adequate fluids and kept under constant one-to-one supervision in a quiet, well-lighted room until transfer to a hospital is arranged. Chlordiazepoxide (Librium®) can be given in doses of 50 to 100 mg by mouth, as needed, for extreme agitation.

B. *Marijuana*—Medical problems attributed to marijuana include acute toxic delirium (acute brain syndrome), usually lasting less than 48 hours, followed by some memory impairment for the episode; or the acute onset of anxiety symptoms and fear, without memory loss or altered sensorium, usually lasting less than 12 hours. Marijuana can also cause chronic bronchitis, chronic nausea or vomiting, headaches, and blackouts, i.e., memory loss for episodes of marijuana intoxication. The above conditions are found more frequently in persons who have used marijuana often for long periods of time.

Signs of marijuana use include the sweet odor of hemp on the breath, reddening of the conjunctivae, increased heart rate, a hearty appetite, a dream-like state of euphoria, and dryness of the throat. High doses cause slurred speech and lack of coordination.

Treatment consists of quiet reassurance and watchful waiting in a quiet place. No medication is indicated.

C. *PCP (phencyclidine, 'angel dust')*—PCP appears in many forms, as a crystalline powder or as tablets and capsules in a variety of colors, shapes, and sizes. It can be inhaled, smoked when sprinkled on parsley or marijuana, swallowed, or injected. It may be mixed with LSD, cocaine, marijuana, or other drugs.

Symptoms include: tachycardia, hypertension, increased deep tendon reflexes, sweating, flushing, drooling, pupillary constriction, dizziness, ataxia, dysarthria, and nystagmus.

Psychological effects are sometimes remarkable and frightening. There may be loss of reality testing, intellectual and emotional disorganization, and a variety of psychotic manifestations. Large doses may lead to coma, seizure, and death.

Acute effects range from a mild loosening of inhibitions to a toxic psychosis, catatonic stupor or excitement, and marked changes in behavior from assaultiveness and uncontrolled belligerence to extreme social withdrawal. Initial symptoms may be similar to amphetamine or cocaine poisoning.

Treatment consists of a quiet, nonstimulating environment. Continuous gastric suction should be started. Diazepam (Valium®) 0.1 to 0.25 mg/kg, given intravenously over a three-minute period, can be used to control convulsions.

For control of violent behavior, haloperidol (Haldol®), 5 mg intramuscularly each hour until the patient is under control, can be used. If restraint is necessary, adequate assistance must be summoned, as a PCP-intoxicated person has unusual strength. Phenothiazines should be withheld until the acute phase has subsided. The patient should be hospitalized in the nearest psychiatric facility.

D. *Hallucinogens*—These include LSD, peyote, and mescaline. Early signs of intoxication are widened pupils, rapid pulse, motor restlessness with hyperreflexia, and sometimes a fine tremor. Blood pressure may be elevated. The patient may complain of vertigo, headache, and nausea. The high period lasts from 8 to 24 hours and may be followed by a low period. The patient's thought processes are markedly disturbed and disorganized, and there is a generalized hyperacuteness of perception. The patient responds to irrelevant stimuli and cannot focus his attention.

Complications of LSD intoxication include bizarre and inappropriate behaviors and occasional severe anxiety or panic states. Suicide and homicide have occurred. Occasionally convulsions occur, and some individuals have prolonged psychotic episodes.

Treatment of the acute phase involves "talking down" and reassurance. Chlorpromazine (Thorazine®), 50 mg intramuscularly, can be given every three to four hours, until the "trip"has subsided.

E. *Anticholinergic alkaloids*—Poisonous plants known for centuries and used as witches' brews are a part of the drug scene. These include belladonna (deadly nightshade), strammonium (Jimson weed or thorn apple), henbane, and angel's trumpet. All four plants contain related anticholinergic alkaloids. Angel's trumpet, which contains scopolamine, is probably the most toxic. If not treated immediately, death may ensue. Scopolamine is found in various over-the-counter medicines, such as Sominex® , Sleep-Eze® , and Compoz® , an overdose of which causes a similar picture of anticholinergic toxicity.

Symptoms include: hot, dry, red skin, increased thirst, widely dilated pupils, increased heart rate, elevated pulse and temperature, drowsiness, hyperactive reflexes, mental confusion, and disorientation for time. Paranoid thinking, slurred speech, and visual and auditory hallucinations may be present.

Treatment consists of slow gastric lavage and the administration of 1 to 4 mg of physostigmine intravenously. Diazepam (Valium®) can be used for quieting the patient. Phenothiazines are contraindicated. Hospitalization in a psychiatric facility should be arranged promptly.

F. *Stimulants*—These include amphetamine, dextroamphetamine, methamphetamine ("speed"), preludin, and cocaine ("coke").

Symptoms of intoxication are: euphoria, hyperactivity, increased speed of thought and speech, loss of appetite, increased alertness, insomnia, irritability, dilated pupils, hyperactive reflexes, and tremor. "Highs" are followed by severe "lows," sometimes leading to suicide. Prolonged usage leads to psychosis, usually paranoid in type. Acute overdose or adverse reaction can lead to convulsions, shock, and death.

Cocaine is a stimulant drug which is being used increasingly. In its various forms it is sniffed, swallowed, smoked, and injected intravenously. Sniffing causes infection, ulceration, and perforation of the nasal septum. Smoking and injecting are the most dangerous and can cause extreme swings from euphoria to deep depression. Consistent use may cause tactile hallucinations and perceptions of something crawling under the skin ("coke bugs"). Ulcerations of the skin can be produced by trying to dig out the "bugs." Visual hallucinations of things in miniature and a picture similar to acute paranoid schizophrenia sometimes occur.

Treatment of acute overdosage consists of diazepam (Valium®) up to 0.25 mg/kg intravenously, physical restraint, if necessary, and transportation to a hospital.

G. *Volatile nitrites ("poppers," "snappers," "locker room")*—The volatile nitrites are used as aphrodisiacs and euphoriants. They are inhaled directly from the bottle or by nasal inhalers, and may be taken in a variety of forms of butyl nitrite.

Symptoms include nausea, dizziness, weakness, tachycardia, flushing, and sometimes fainting. Pulsating headaches frequently occur. The effects are usually brief in duration. Long-term usage may lead to the development of methemoglobinemia.

Treatment is symptomatic, but recognition of the possible cause of the typical symptoms is important.

H. *Barbiturates and other sedatives*—The short-acting barbiturates such as Seconal® or Nembutal®, and sleep medications such as Placidyl®, Doriden®, and Quaalude® are the most frequently used sedative-type drugs. Symptoms of intoxication range from somnolence to coma.

Emergency measures for the comatose patient include immediate attention to the airway with endotracheal intubation with cuff inflated if the patient will tolerate it. The patient should be ventilated using positive pressure and compressed air at a rate of 10-12/minute.

The blood pressure should be checked and an infusion of dextrose and water or normal saline started through a large-gauge needle. A blood specimen (10 ml, clotted) should be taken for laboratory tests.

Look for evidence of trauma in addition to specific signs of intoxication. Record all physical findings and procedures carefully, and arrange for transfer to a hospital.

Barbiturate withdrawal syndrome may occur shortly after a person's arrival at camp. Usually a careful history will reveal the use of short-acting barbiturates in doses of 1500 mg/day or more. Withdrawal can be life-threatening and requires hospitalization. If seizures have developed, emergency treatment with 100 to 200 mg of phenobarbital intramuscularly can be given while hospitalization is arranged.

A Note on Hospitalization

Each state has laws governing admission to psychiatric hospitals. A camp physician should have the names of two or three nearby psychiatrists who can act as consultants or referral sources when needed. As with any medical emergency, a psychiatric emergency necessitates notification of nearest of kin. Telephone permissions for emergency treatment, if witnessed by two listeners, are generally accepted.

References

Diagnostic and Statistical Manual of Mental Disorders (Third Edition). "DSM III" American Psychiatric Association, 1980.

Klein, D. F., Gittelman, R., Quitkin, F., Rifkin, A. *Diagnosis and Drug Treatment of Psychiatric Disorders, Adults and Children.* 2nd Edition, Williams & Wilkins, Baltimore, 1980.

Bourne, P.G. *Acute Drug Abuse Emergencies; A Treatment Manual.* Academic Press, N.Y., 1976.

"Drug Abuse: A Guide for the Primary Care Physician." AMA Order Dept., OP-323, P.O. Box 821, Monroe, Wisc., 53566, 1981.

Gabel, S. (Ed.), *Behavioral Problems in Childhood: A Primary Care Approach.* Grune & Stratten, N.Y., 1981.

Dubin, W. R. and Stolberg, R. *Emergency Psychiatry for the House Officer.* Spectrum Publications, N.Y., 1981 (paperback).

Stewart, M. A. and Gath, A. *Psychological Disorders of Children: A Handbook for Primary Care Physicians.* Williams & Wilkins, Baltimore, 1978.

Norris, A. S. *Psychopharmacology for Primary Physicians.* Charles C. Thomas, Springfield, Ill., 1981.

Chapter VI

CAMPING AND THE HANDICAPPED CHILD

Most physicians, parents, and camp directors would agree that a handicapped child should not be deprived of the camping experience. There may be disagreement as to whether the handicapped child should attend a special camp which is geared to his particular handicap or whether it would be best for the child to be "mainstreamed" in a regular camp.

Some specific handicapping disorders which require careful consideration are: diabetes, blindness, deafness, cystic fibrosis, mental retardation, and crippling orthopedic or neurologic disorders. With the above handicaps certain emergencies may arise which the camp personnel must be aware of and know how to treat. For example, a diabetic may have a "fainting" spell because of low blood sugar, and need sugar, plus an adjustment of his insulin dosage. The child with cystic fibrosis is at risk of fainting and collapse, especially in hot weather, because of a low sodium concentration in the blood. The blind, deaf, mentally retarded, orthopedically or neurologically handicapped child will need close supervision requiring an increase in the number of trained staff members.

Camps which specialize in programs for children with specific handicapping conditions necessarily have the equipment and personnel to handle the medical, physical, and social needs of these children. If a regular camp accepts a number of campers with any of the above handicaps, certain requirements must be met so that the handicapped child is not placed at an unacceptable risk and is able to participate as fully as possible in the program. These include counselors with specialized training relevant to the handicapping condition. One trained counselor could teach and supervise others who would be involved in the child's care. A full-time registered nurse and/or physician would be required. In addition, some necessary physical changes would have to be made in the camp facilities, such as installation of ramps, special toilets, and special dining facilities, in order to meet the requirements of some handicapped children.

If a camp has the facilities and the personnel, on what basis can the decision be made to accept or reject a handicapped child? In general, if a child has been mainstreamed successfully in school, then one would expect that he could benefit by a camp experience with non-handicapped children. Such a handicapped child could provide a valuable experience in sharing and caring for the non-handicapped children.

If school mainstreaming has never been attempted or was unsuccessful, then the decision is more difficult. Would the camp experience help this child to make a better adjustment in school? Does the camp have the capability in terms of staff expertise to provide for this child's special needs and to promote a healthy experience? Is this camp a safe place for this child? Would having this child in camp enhance or interfere with the camp experience of the other children? Parents of a handicapped child deserve thoughtful answers to the above questions.

Before rejecting an application on the basis of handicap, two alternative possibilities might be considered. One, a handicapped child who lives within easy traveling distance of the camp might be admitted on a part-time basis to participate in activities which seem most appropriate.

A second option to consider is having an understanding older child "caregiver" attend the camp as companion and tutor for the handicapped child, for his protection and guidance. This might be helpful, for instance, for a blind, deaf, or crippled child whose only opportunity for camping lies in a regular camp.

If the decision is favorable toward admitting a handicapped child, what steps could be taken to enhance the experience psychologically for all the children? First of all the camp doctor should inform the other staff members of the child's condition and how to handle emergencies.

Second, it would be very important to learn from the parents as much as possible about their handicapped child. Helpful information would include: the extent of the child's independence, the parents' methods of care, what the child is like as a person, how he usually gets along with his peers, whether he has friends, what he enjoys doing, what his best skills are, and what activities, if any, should be avoided.

On the first day, the camp physician should become personally acquainted with the child by observing him in the various activities and situations. A very outgoing, confident child in a wheelchair may make his own way with peers without adult help. However, if the child is shy or sensitive, or has been the subject of either ridicule or neglect in the past, special efforts will be needed to help him find his place in camp.

To assist with this, a group meeting with his cabin or tent mates to answer their questions, and to get their ideas about how their handicapped member may be integrated into cabin and camp life will be helpful. When a matter is put before them, children will often come up with good ideas adults might not think of. The emphasis should be on understanding, caring, and sharing.

One should try to avoid totally one-sided arrangements whereby one camper takes over a handicapped child and becomes the sole protector and guide. A better plan would be the scheduling of taking turns in guiding, going with, or helping at different times of the day with various functions. In this way the handicapped child will get to know more campers and more children will benefit from the experience of helping and sharing. The exception would be the hired "caregiver" plan described previously. Even then, other children should be encouraged to share their time and activities as appropriate.

Handicapping conditions vary a lot in the degree of independence which the condition affords. A blind child, for instance, needs more guidance and protection in a new setting than a deaf child. However, many handicapped persons like to be as independent as possible and are disturbed when attention is drawn to the handicap. The art of assisting when needed without smothering is one which the non-handicapped have to learn. Some children learn this on their own. They quickly pick up cues from the handicapped and react with sensitivity and grace. Others need more concrete instruction and modelling in their efforts to help. The Health Supervisor may be able to act as model and instructor for camp adults and children alike when situations requiring special sensitivity arise.

Neurological Disorders

As examples of children with handicaps who might be "mainstreamed" are those with selected neurological disorders and diabetes.

A. Seizure Disorder

A child may experience a seizure if already on anticonvulsant medication or may have his first seizure while at camp.

The management of convulsive seizures (also known as generalized tonic-clonic or grand mal convulsions) is as follows. Protect the child by placing something soft under the head as a cushion. Remove any sharp or dangerous objects from the area. Do not restrain the child or force anything into the mouth. Turn the child onto his side to allow drainage of food and saliva from the mouth and to keep the airway clear. Do not give anything to eat or drink until fully awake. Stay with the child until the seizure ends. Give artificial respiration if breathing does not resume after the seizure ends. Be reassuring and allow the child to rest for an hour or so afterwards in a supervised setting. The seizure will usually last a short time; however, if a second seizure occurs shortly after the first, or if a seizure lasts much longer than 10 minutes, referred to as *status epileipticus* or "non-stop" seizures, the person should be taken to a medical facility immediately, especially one where expert neurologic consultation is available. If a camper is taken to a hospital, the parents should be notified and given an account of the incident and given reassurance that the child is well cared for.

If a child who is not known to have epilepsy experiences a convulsive seizure for the first time, the treatment should be outlined as above. In such a case, the condition may be caused by some underlying infection or metabolic problem. The parents should be notified and the camper should be taken to the nearest medical facility where competent consultation is available.

Non-convulsive seizures may take the form of brief staring spells, automatic behavior with altered consciousness, or involuntary movements of an arm or leg. No first aid procedures are required for seizures involving brief staring spells or involuntary movements of the limbs. However, if a child has an episode of *automatic behavior*, the counselor should guide the child gently away from hazards and stay with the child until full consciousness returns.

Another type of neurologic disorder may be the "drop-attack," also called atonic or akinetic seizures. Drop attacks produce sudden and complete loss of muscle tone, causing the child to drop to the ground—sometimes with considerable force. Children subject to this type of seizure should wear some form of helmet to prevent injury to the head.

Compliance with medication is extremely important in a child with epilepsy and should be checked carefully. A sudden interruption of medication may lead to an increase in the number of seizures. It is strongly advised that the medication be kept in the infirmary and that the nurse administer the medication to assure compliance. If a camper goes on a three or four day trip, the nurse should give the counselor in charge the medication with instructions on how and when to administer the medicine. The Health Supervisor should have on file a complete medical summary on any known epileptic as well as a detailed account about the administration of the medication.

If a camper has a seizure, it is important to explain to the other campers the nature of epilepsy in simple terms and give them a chance to talk about what happened and ask questions. This will calm their fears and reduce anxiety. The Health Supervisor should assure the other campers that epilepsy is not contagious. The other campers should also be reassured that the camper with the seizure is no threat to them and is no different from the other campers and that the seizures will usually be controlled with medicine. The reaction of fear is understandable and discussing this with the campers in a quiet, unemotional manner will transform a potentially disruptive event into a learning experience.

In most cases, the child with epilepsy will have sufficient seizure control on medication and will benefit from regular camping activities. The camper should be able to do so without special limitations. In any case, the child with epilepsy should be watched carefully in any situation in which sudden loss of consciousness or altered consciousness might pose a hazard to the child, such as swimming and horseback riding.

The preceding information was taken from a booklet which has been developed by the Epilepsy Foundation of America* and is available upon request. It is strongly urged that the camp director make this available to the Health Supervisor in charge as well as the counseling staff if a camp is willing to take children with epilepsy as campers.

B. Specific Developmental Disorders

An otherwise normal child may have a developmental reading or language disorder, the former usually referred to as a learning disability or dyslexia, and the latter as either dysphasia or an aphasia.

---

*Epilepsy Foundation of America, 4351 Garden City Drive, Landover, MD 20785

Reading disability becomes important at camp if the activities involve reading and if the child is subjected to ridicule or embarrassment when the disability becomes apparent. Difficulties in speaking can likewise be a source of great embarrassment for a child who has a speech or language problem.

An understanding Health Supervisor can be helpful in adjustment problems which arise related to these difficulties. Education of the staff and campers about the nature of the difficulty may be important in helping the child to cope better with the problem.

C. Pervasive Developmental Disorders

A mildly autistic child who has been in regular school classes might also attend a regular camp. Such a child may have unique ways of verbalizing and socializing, may use language inappropriately, may be concrete in thinking, may have odd mannerisms, and may be rather awkward socially. Often the autistic young person is uninhibited in verbal expression and lacks a sense of social propriety. These characteristics can lead to ridicule, embarrassment, and isolation.

A careful medical history will reveal difficulties from very early in life. Clarification of the nature of the condition will help counselors to integrate such a child into the camp program and prevent the social ostracism which might otherwise occur.

D. Mildly Organic Children

This includes a heterogenous group of children, often loosely diagnosed as having non-specific brain dysfunction. The etiology, if known, may be related to perinatal difficulties, head trauma, or serious illness affecting the central nervous system. The child may or may not have a seizure disorder or hyperkinesis.

These children stand out among their peers because of the following characteristics: being irritable, moody, easily upset, impulsive, uninhibited, and concrete in their thinking. They usually are slow learners in some areas, average to bright in others. They overreact to changes in routine and to the unexpected. Judgment and insight are often impaired. They may display an unusual amount of oppositional behavior, i.e., temper tantrums, argumentativeness, and stubborn resistance to instruction.

A Health Supervisor who understands the problem can be helpful to counselors and other staff in working with an organically impaired camper. Patience, close supervision, and supportive encouragement are essential. These children respond best to a well-structured program and a regular daily routine.

Diabaetes Mellitus in Adolescents and Children*

Insulin-dependent diabetes mellitus is a disease manifest by severe metabolic imbalance which is a result of insulin deficiency. Treatment consists of a well-balanced program of insulin administration, diet, and exercise. Improper balance of these three elements of therapy can result in hyperglycemia (high blood sugar), hypoglycemia (low blood sugar), or the severe metabolic derangement known as diabetic ketoacidosis.

Insulin

All insulin-dependent diabetic subjects (this includes nearly all children and adolescents with diabetes) require insulin administration as part of their therapy. Oral hypoglycemic agents, such as tolbutamide or chlorpropramide, are not useful in managing diabetic children. Insulin must be given as injections. Insulin injections are usually given as a mixture of a short-acting insulin (Regular) and intermediate-acting insulin (NPH or Lente). These are usually mixed in a single syringe and given subcutaneously as one or two injections per day, usually before breakfast and supper. Recently, more intensive regimens of insulin delivery have been initiated in some patients; these include 3-5 injections per day or a continuous subcutaneous insulin infusion via a portable infusion pump. However, currently, these more aggressive modes of therapy are used by less than 10 percent of adolescents with diabetes mellitus.

Insulin is available as preparations of varying purity and from multiple species, including beef, pork, and human. Most preparations currently in use contain 100 units of insulin per cc (U-100). Insulin syringes are specific for the concentration of insulin used; that is, U-100 insulin should be administered *only* using a U-100 insulin syringe. If a mixture of two different kinds of insulin is to be given at the same time, they can be mixed in a single syringe and given as a single injection. This mixing should take place as soon before the injection as possible. Insulin injections should be given 15-30 minutes before the meal, but the timing can vary depending on the subject. Some diabetic subjects vary the time of the injection depending on blood sugar.

Insulin is stable in solution for extended periods of time (check expiration date on vial). Although no special handling or storage is needed, exposure to either freezing or high temperatures should be avoided.

Diet

The diet of a diabetic child is a well-balanced meal plan calculated to supply adequate nutrition and calories for normal growth and develop-

---

*This section was written by Neil H. White, M.D., Assistant Professor of Pediatrics, Washington University School of Medicine.

ment. The specific dietary prescription must be individualized and depends on age, sex, body weight, level of activity, and other factors. Normal growth and development and maintenance of ideal body weight should be maintained, and obesity should be avoided. Although the caloric intake is usually not restricted, it is often calculated. The meal plan is designed to achieve as little day-to-day variation in quantity, composition, and distribution of food as possible. Meal plans for insulin-dependent diabetics usually consist of three meals per day, along with one to three snacks. For diabetic subjects who take morning insulin as a mixture of Regular and NPH or Lente, the timing of meals is critical. Breakfast needs to be eaten shortly (15-60 minutes) after the insulin dose, and lunch should be four or five hours later. Otherwise hypoglycemia (as a result of NPH insulin) is likely. For those using multiple doses of regular insulin before eating or an insulin pump, there can be more flexibility of the timing of meals. However, this only accounts for a small proportion of children and adolescents with diabetes. A bedtime snack is nearly always recommended. During sustained increased levels of activity, as at camp, an increase in the caloric content of the meal plan or additional snack is often needed.

Exercise

The effects of exercise on metabolism are complex. In the presence of insulin, exercise lowers blood sugar. However, in the face of insulin deficiency, exercise raises blood sugar. Therefore, diabetic persons who plan to engage in strenuous physical activity must remember two points:

1) exercise only when in adequate control (blood sugar below 250 mg/dl and no ketones), not when poorly controlled (blood sugar over 300 mg/dl with or without ketones);
2) when exercising, be alert to the possibility of hypoglycemia. Exercise after a meal can reduce postprandial hyperglycemia; however, exercise before breakfast and morning insulin can result in preprandial hyperglycemia.

Hyperglycemia

Hyperglycemia, or high blood sugar, can result from insufficient insulin, improperly timed insulin dose, excess carbohydrate intake, insufficient exercise, stress, or infection. Hyperglycemia is detected either by the meaurement of a high blood sugar or by the presence of glycosuria (glucose in the urine). Glycosuria usually occurs only if blood glucose is over 180-200 mg/dl. This is called the renal threshold. Hyperglycemia and glycosuria are responsible for the well-known symptoms of diabetes, namely polyuria, polydipsia, and nocturia. Marked hyperglycemia resulting in symptoms should be avoided. However, the long-term effects of lesser degrees of hyperglycemia are unknown.

Hypoglycemia

Hypoglycemia, or low blood sugar, can result from excess insulin, reduced dietary intake, or an increased level of physical activity. Mild hypoglycemia consists of symptoms such as sweating, shakiness, severe hunger, and fast heart rate. These are "adrenergic" symptoms, meaning they are a result of adrenalin release. These symptoms serve as a warning that hypoglycemia is present or approaching, not as a sign of danger. These mild hypoglycemic episodes, or insulin reactions, are a common feature of well-controlled diabetes mellitus, and often occur before meals or during exercise. The total absence of bouts of mild hypoglycemia often indicates persistent hyperglycemia. Mild hypoglycemia should be treated by the ingestion of 5-15 grams of carbohydrate. If there is no improvement in 20 minutes, this should be repeated. One packet of sugar contains 4 grams, one "Lifesaver" contains 2 grams, and 4 ounces (1/2 cup) of orange juice contains 10 grams of carbohydrate.

Severe hypoglycemia consists of a low blood sugar resulting in unconsciousness, seizure, or any form of reduced mental status. This represents a potential medical emergency and thus requires immediate attention. Severe hypoglycemia, often called insulin shock, should be treated either with intravenous glucose (10-20 gm Dextrose) or intramuscular glucagon (0.5-1.0 gm). Oral carbohydrate should be given when alert, and the subject should be carefully observed for a recurrence of hypoglycemia over the next few hours. The reason for a severe hypoglycemic episode should be sought.

Monitoring

In addition to the carefully regulated regimen of insulin, diet, and exercise, diabetic subjects must constantly monitor their disease. Monitoring is usually done before meals using urine tests toglycosuria (Clinitest, DiaStix, and others), or using glucose oxidase reagent strips (Dextrostix or BG Chemstrips) to measure blood glucose. The blood sample is obtained from the finger by needle prick after washing the hands with soap and water, followed by wiping the area to be punctured with 70 percent alcohol. Self blood glucose monitoring has become more popular over the last few years. Appropriate blood sugar goals must be set for each individual, but in general, recurrent hypoglycemia (less than 50 mg/dl) or hyperglycemia (greater than 250 mg/dl) results in symptoms, reduced energy, and a reduced feeling of well-being. If only blood sugars are being monitored, urine needs to be checked for ketones when blood sugar is high or during illness. The presence of moderate or large ketonuria usually indicates metabolic imbalance and requires more aggressive intervention.

Intercurrent Illness and Sick Day Management in Diabetes Mellitus

Any form of infection or stress increases the insulin requirements. This is true for mild illness such as a "cold" or the "flu," as well as for serious illness. Larger or additional doses of insulin (usually given as Regular insulin) are often needed to prevent hyperglycemia and ketosis during illness. Fever, hyperglycemia, vomiting, and diarrhea may result in dehydration. Thus, an increased fluid intake is needed during illness. In addition, in the face of the larger doses of insulin needed to prevent hyperglycemia and ketosis, hypoglycemia may occur. Ingestion of carbohydrate-containing fluids may be indicated. In general, two to three ounces of additional fluid every 30-45 minutes is usually a good goal, but more may be needed for larger subjects or if ongoing fluid losses are large. If oral intake is impossible, either because of vomiting or other intercurrent illness, intravenous fluid along with insulin is often needed to prevent diabetic ketoacidosis (DKA). DKA is a severe metabolic imbalance manifest by dehydration, ketosis, acidosis, hyperglycemia, and Kussmaul respiration (deep, labored breathing). Treatment of DKA usually requires intravenous fluid therapy and medical attention in a setting where close monitoring and access to a laboratory is available. Hospitalization is required.

Summary

The diabetic child or adolescent can lead an essentially normal life without any restrictions on activities. However, attention must be paid to the medical regimen including insulin, diet, exercise, and monitoring. The day-to-day adherence to this regimen is primarily the responsibility of the diabetic subject and his or her family, but those responsible for the care of a diabetic child must be aware of the symptoms and signs of hypoglycemia and ketoacidosis and should be aware of the procedures needed to treat these or acquire the necessary medical help. If a camp accepts diabetic children as campers, the camp director must insist upon a complete medical summary about the camper with complete instructions about the medical care of the camper. The insulin injections and the testing of urine and blood for sugar content should be done in the infirmary under the observation of the Health Supervisor. If the camper leaves camp for two or three days, the Health Supervisor must instruct the counselor in charge about the administration of insulin and the monitoring of sugar tests of the blood and urine. It would also be advisable for the camp physician and/or nurse to have concise informational booklets about diabetes mellitus which may be obtained from the following organizations:

American Diabetes Association
600 Fifth Avenue
New York, NY 10020

Juvenile Diabetes Foundation
23 East 26th Street
New York, NY 10010

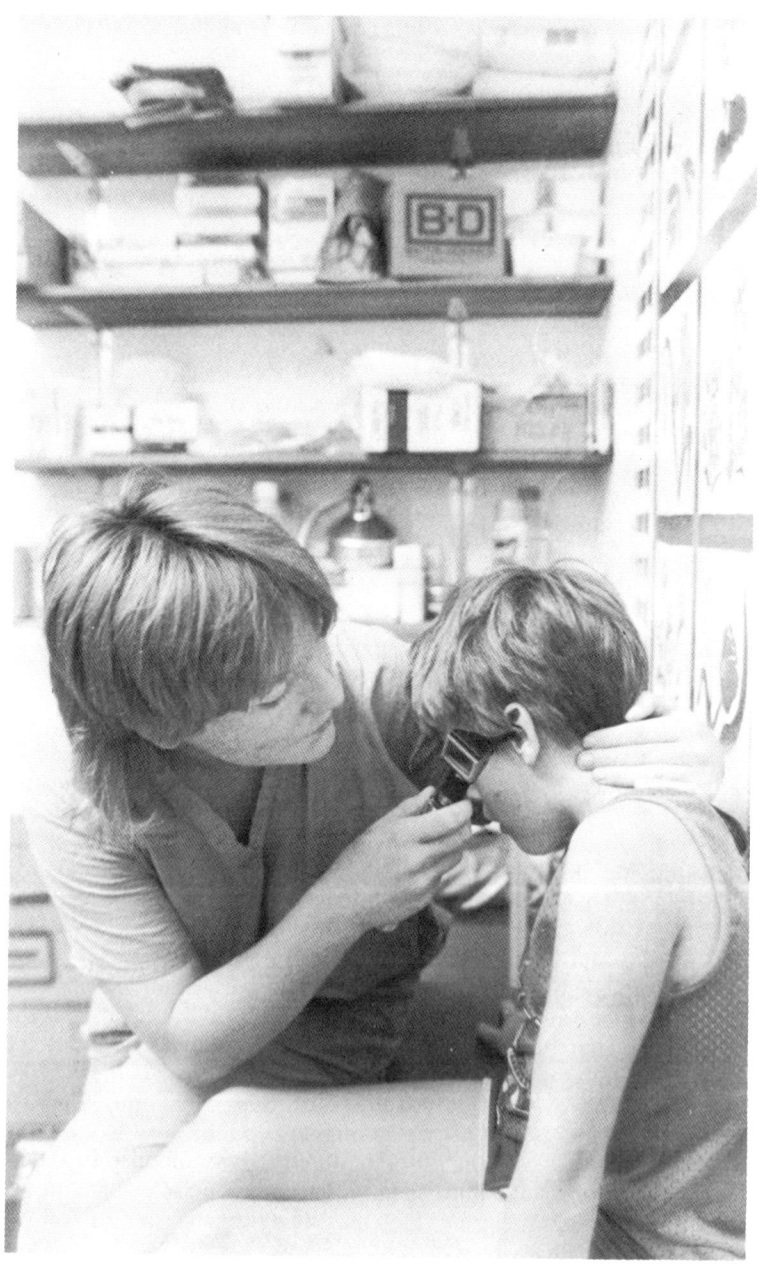

Chapter VII

EAR, NOSE, THROAT, AND CHEST PROBLEMS

Upper and lower respiratory infections are seen with great frequency at camp. The counseling staff should be instructed carefully about the importance of seeking medical aid when a camper shows evidence of a respiratory infection. This will insure prompt treatment and possibly prevent the spread of infection. The respiratory infection may manifest itself by a stuffy or runny nose, a cough, hoarseness, or complaints of sore throat or earache. The Health Supervisor should check the camper's temperature, and if he is febrile, he should be admitted to the infirmary for one to two days of observation and treatment. If a camper's complaints are minimal, he might be allowed to return to his cabin, but he should be restricted from swimming until he is free of complaints or symptoms.

The Health Supervisor must be aware that it is unusual to encounter serious respiratory infections in a camp setting, and with the large spectrum of potent antibiotic medication now available, most bacterial infections are quickly brought under control. It is important to realize that bacteria are no longer recognized as the prime offenders. A host of viruses have been discovered which account for many of the respiratory infections. The anatomic areas involved by the infections are the nose, throat, larynx, trachea, and bronchi. In recent years a number of viruses have been reported as the cause of acute upper and lower respiratory infections. Infectious viruses associated with the common cold include over 100 different rhinoviruses, four parainfluenza, respiratory syncytial, many coronaviruses, over 30 adenoviruses, 24 Coxsackie A, six Coxsackie B, 32 ECHO, and three Reoviruses, in addition to the three known influenza agents.

Pharyngoconjunctival fever is primarily associated with adenovirus type three but types one through eight and 14 have also been observed in association with this disease.

Herpangina, with its papules, vesicles, and ulcerative lesions involving the uvula, soft palate, tonsils, tonsillar pillars, and occasionally the posterior pharynx, is associated primarily with Coxsackie A, B, and ECHO viruses.

It is important to realize that viruses may be responsible for most mild epidemics of respiratory infections at camp. It is equally important to realize that it is quite difficult to make an accurate diagnosis clinically and differentiate with confidence between bacterial and viral infections. It has been our practice to institute antibiotic therapy and observe the patient, especially if there is appreciable fever and toxicity. Most camps are near enough to a state health laboratory so that a throat culture can be obtained and the presence of Group A beta hemolytic streptococci can be ruled out. The result of the culture, however, may not be received for two to three days, and it is best to treat with antibiotics before a diagnosis is made, especially if the index of suspicion is high that a camper may have a streptococcal infection. If the organism is the streptococcus or pneumococcus, quick institution of antibiotic therapy will quickly return the camper to activity. If, on the other hand, the febrile respiratory infection is of one to two days duration and seems unaffected by antibiotic therapy, the other campers who develop the infection may be treated symptomatically. There may be some criticism because of the over-enthusiastic use of antibiotics, but in a camp situation we feel that this is justified. The risk involved in the use of antibiotics is probably less than the risk of allowing a streptococcal, pheumococcal, or staphylococcal infection to go untreated for two to three days. Since one cannot identify the bacterial agent, a broad-spectrum antibiotic should be the one of choice.

Again, it is worthwhile to reemphasize—if an upper or lower respiratory infection seems unaffected by drug therapy and the camper shows no improvement in two to three days, it is best to consider hospitalization where adequate facilities are available.

Nosebleed

This is a fairly common event, especially in a boys' camp, and is usually caused by trauma. If this should happen away from camp, the camper should be made to rest in a semi-erect position. Cold applications to the bridge of the nose may help. Firm compression of the tip of the nose with the forefinger and the thumb may also help. The bleeding usually stops in one or two minutes.

The camper should be taken to the infirmary. An examination will reveal the site and extent of the hemorrhage. If packing is necessary, the camper should be transferred to a hospital unless the camp Health Supervisor has had experience in this area. Causes other than trauma should be kept in mind; examples are congestion resulting from a foreign body, hypertrophied adenoids, or allergy. Varicosities and telangiectases of the mucous membrane of the anterior septum may be a cause. Epistaxis due to hypertension, blood dyscrasias, and rheumatic fever should be kept in mind. Normal saline nose drops (six to eight drops in each nostril four times daily) and gentle application of vaseline to the lower septum with a fingertip may prevent recurrences.

Acute External Otitis (Swimmer's Ear)

This condition may follow trauma or swimming in contaminated water. Sometimes it is due to mechanical probing in an effort to clean the external auditory canal.

The camper will complain of earache, and there may be a discharge from the ear canal, pain on movement of the ear, and redness and swelling of the external auditory canal. Other findings include pruritis, scaling, hearing loss, and fullness.

Warm wet packs give relief, and the use of eardrops such as Auralgan® may give some relief. Aspirin or acetaminophen will help relieve the pain. The camper should be restricted from swimming. This type of infection should be seen and treated by a physician.

The cause usually is bacterial. In 75-90 percent of the cases, the predominant organism is *Pseudomonas aeruginosa.* Other organisms isolated are *Staphylococcus epidermidis, Proteus mirabilis, Klebsiella pneumoniae,* and *Escherichia coli.*

The principles of treatment include (a) thorough cleansing of the external auditory canal, (b) acidification, (c) judicious limited use of antibiotic medication, (d) relief of pain and discomfort, (e) elimination or control of predisposing causes (i.e., keep all water out of the ear and forbid swimming). These principles entail the suctioning or cleaning of debris from the external auditory canal. Acid preparations for instillation or irrigation include Otic Demboro®, VoSol Otic®, or VoSol HC Otic® solutions. Specific medications containing antibiotics that can be instilled are Corticosporin otic solution or suspension® and Coly-Mycin S Otic®. Chloromycetin Otic® is useful in patients allergic to neomycin. These contain antibiotics that inhibit multiplication of surface bacteria and prevent invasion. The introduction of a wick into the external auditory canal may help distribution of the medication if the canal is edematous.

Severe cases where cellulitis, lymphadenopathy, or systemic infection are present may be caused by bacteria (staphylococcus or streptococcus). Treatment with oral antibiotics (ampicillin, amoxicillin, cephalosporin) is indicated. It is wise to get the help of a consultant if the infection does not show evidence of improvement in several days. This is particularly true for the camper with diabetes mellitus. When vesiculation of the external canal occurs, the cause is usually the Herpes simplex virus. The pain is severe, and the treatment should be symptomatic.

Hemorrhagic blebs are usually caused by viral infections. Relief may be obtained by rupturing the blebs with a cotton applicator. The camper should be restricted from swimming, although showers may be taken.

Acute Otitis Media

This is an infection of the middle ear and is usually secondary to an upper respiratory infection. The camper complains of earache and is febrile. The external ear shows no abnormality, but pulling upon the ear will cause pain. The camper should be seen by a physician, and until then, an ice bag and aspirin will give some relief. The nurse should not instill ear drops, because this will obscure the landmarks of the tympanic membrane. After the physician has seen the patient, symptomatic relief can be achieved by instilling Auralgan®. The specific treatment, however, is the administration of oral antibiotics (penicillin, amoxicillin, or

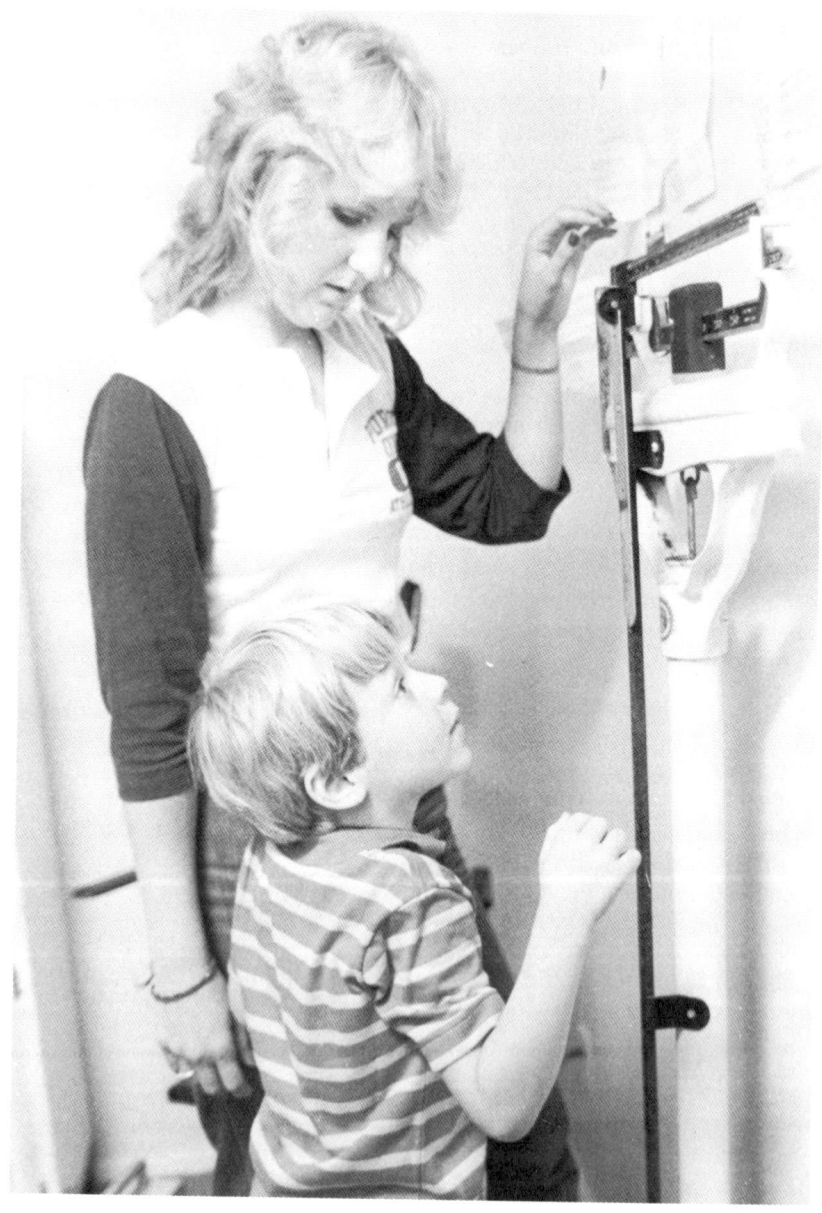

erythromycin-sulfonamide combinations for those allergic to penicillin). Usually 10-14 days of treatment are necessary, and the camper should be examined every day and restricted from swimming until the infection has cleared.

Chronic Otitis Media

Chronic otitis media is relatively rare. If an acute otitis media persists for three to six weeks after adequate antibiotic therapy, one should suspect mastoiditis. A problem of this nature cannot be handled in camp, and the patient should be sent home. On rare occasions the Health Supervisor sees perforated eardrums in camp. Acute perforation of the eardrum usually occurs from indirect trauma such as a blow with the open palm, severe head injuries, and concussion from an explosion. The perforation is followed immediately by bleeding, pain, and hearing impairment. The canal should be kept closed with sterile cotton, and a prophylactic antibiotic is indicated to prevent infection. No liquid ear drops should be instilled. The perforation will usually heal spontaneously. Of course, swimming should be prohibited until the perforation is healed. Expert consultation from an ear, nose, and throat specialist should be sought to guide the camp physician, especially if severe hearing loss or vertigo is present. Trauma sufficient to rupture an eardrum may cause other injuries, so complete evaluation and close observation are important.

Foreign Bodies in the Ear

Various animate and inanimate foreign bodies may be introduced into the external auditory canal. Unless these are visible, within easy reach, and the camper cooperative, it is best to remove them under general anesthesia in a hospital. Irrigation of particles should be avoided since absorption of water may increase their size. A few drops of ether will anesthetize insects so they can be removed; alcohol tends to stimulate furious activity before the insect dies.

Cerumen may become inspissated and impacted. A small mass of cerumen may be removed by *gentle* and *careful* extraction with a hook or curette. If one is not experienced, this should not be attempted. If removal of the cerumen is absolutely necessary, large masses should be softened with the installation of Debrox® or Cerumenex®. These may then be removed by irrigation with warm water.

Foreign Bodies in the Nose

This type of accident has not been encountered in my years of camping, but the introduction of foreign bodies such as peas, cherry stones, or beads into the nose may occur. The foreign body is usually situated well forward unless efforts by the patient or an unskilled physician pack it backwards.

The early symptoms are obstruction to respiration, pain, and sneezing. If the foreign body is nonreactive, it may be lodged in the nose for weeks without producing marked symptoms. Usually there is enough irritation so that secondary infection takes place, and the patient has a serosanguineous or purulent discharge; this in itself should arouse suspicion. A careful examination will usually help make the diagnosis, and removal of the foreign body is best accomplished away from camp by an ear, nose, and throat specialist.

Chapter VIII

SKIN PROBLEMS

by Thomas W. Cooper, M.D.
Instructor in Medicine in Dermatology, Division of Dermatology
Department of Internal Medicine
Washington University School of Medicine

Most children or camp personnel with chronic skin diseases have been diagnosed and specific therapy begun prior to their arriving at camp. These diseases should be noted on the camper's health form as well as the specific treatment recommended by their physician. The dermatological problems commonly encountered at camp may include all of the following.

Sunburn

The frequency of sunburn is greatest in early summer and during the first few weeks of camp. In a fair-complexioned individual, the minimal erythema dose is approximately 15 minutes of noonday sun at 40 degrees latitude north. Four to eight times this dose will produce moderate to severe sunburn reaction. A mild sunburn reaction usually causes a feeling of tenderness and tautness of the skin. Severe reactions may be intensely painful and associated with nausea, fever, and tachycardia. Within the first two to four hours of exposure, the skin is pink and slightly edematous. The maximal response is seen at approximately 18 hours when the skin is intensely erythematous, edematous, and may progress to blistering.

Mild sunburn can be treated with cool tapwater compresses for 20 minutes three times a day to the affected areas. Topical steroid in lotion or cream may reduce inflammation. Emollients such as Eucerin® or Lubriderm® will relieve dryness. Aspirin or other prostaglandin inhibitors by mouth may also be given for symptomatic relief. Severe sunburn may be treated using the above measures. In addition, systemic corticosteroids may attenuate a severe sunburn response if given early. The equivalent of 60 mg prednisone in an adult should be given orally each day for three days and then stopped.

Prevention of sunburn is obviously preferable to treatment and should be stressed to the counselors by the camp physician and camp director during the indoctrination sessions before the camping session. Prevention of sunburn includes avoidance of midday sun, protective clothing, use of sunscreens containing para-aminobenzoic acid (PABA), and application of opaque substances such as zinc oxide ointment. PABA-containing sunscreens have a sun protection factor ranging from minimal protection of a grade number of 2-3 to almost complete protection of 15. Those individuals with fair skin need to be especially careful, because they are subject not only to acute sun damage, but also to chronic changes such a premature aging and malignant degeneration of the skin.

Poison Ivy Dermatitis

This condition is commonly seen during the camping season. Counselors should be familiar with the plant *Rhus radicans* which causes poison ivy dermatitis. This plant may be a climbing or a trailing vine or erect bush which may reach a height of four feet. Sensitization and dermatitis will occur in 70 percent of individuals who come in contact with the oily resin released by a crushed portion of the plant. Animals, clothing, shoes, and gloves can be contaminated with the resin, making it possible for an individual to develop dermatitis without direct plant contact.

A very sensitive individual may develop dermatitis in 6-12 hours if there has been intense exposure to the plant, but usually the rash appears in one to three days. The primary symptom is pruritus, but discomfort related to dryness and pain due to vesicles and ulcers may also occur. The typical physical findings of plant dermatitis are linear and grouped vesicles and bullae. If the reaction is severe, edema and erythema may be prominent, particularly in the periorbital and genital areas. Palms, soles, and scalp show relative resistance to contact dermatitis. The lesions tend to clear in one to three weeks, depending on the severity of the eruption. The vesicle fluid is a tissue transudate of body fluid and will *not* spread the dermatitis to other areas on the body or to other people.

If an individual comes in contact with the poison ivy plant or if acute plant dermatitis is diagnosed, he should wash thoroughly. For a mild eruption, the following steps will provide symptomatic relief: (a) cool Burow's solution (5 percent aluminum acetate diluted 1:20) or saline compresses lasting 20 minutes four times a day (b) Lubriderm® lotion containing 1/4 percent menthol and 1 percent phenol applied two to four times a day, (c) topical steroid, (d) antihistamines. For widespread eruption, tepid tub baths may also provide symptomatic relief. If the rash is severe enough and no contraindications are present, systemic steroids may be employed. Prednisone in a dose starting at about 0.8 mg/kg is appropriate. The dose should be gradually tapered over two or three weeks. If the course is any shorter, the underlying inflammatory reaction may recur when corticosteroids are stopped. Secondary infections should be treated with systemic antibiotics. Desensitization procedures have not been particularly effective and are not recommended. The most important preventive measures are avoiding the poison ivy and poison oak plants and, if possible, ridding campgrounds of these offending weeds.

Abrasions

Abrasions should be cleaned thoroughly with soap and water. Application of Betadine® ointment and a bandage will often prevent secondary infection. If infection occurs, soaking the affected area for 20 minutes four times a day in warm water and application of Polysporin® ointment will usually clear up the infection. If the infected area does not respond to this therapy in two to three days, if fever develops, or if the area of redness enlarges, systemic antibiotics are probably indicated. Erythromycin and dicloxicillin are both effective agents (see Impetigo for dosage). Tetanus immunization status should be determined and tetanus immune globulin and/or toxoid administered if indicated (see *Table V*).

Foreign Body

Splinters and other foreign bodies frequently become embedded in the skin. If the foreign body cannot be easily removed, then the superficial skin can be shaved, enabling the foreign body to be removed with fine, sterile tweezers. A magnifying glass will often help visualize a small foreign body, and glass can often be felt if it cannot be seen. After the foreign body is removed, the area should be washed thoroughly with soap and water and Betadine® ointment should be applied. If secondary infection occurs, systemic antibiotics should be given. Tetanus immunization status should be determined and tetanus immune globulin and/or toxoid administered if indicated (see *Table V*).

Blisters

Loose-fitting shoes and unaccustomed use of hand tools and athletic equipment may lead to friction blisters. Small blisters can be covered with a Band-aid® while the fluid slowly resorbs. If the blister is large and prone to rupture, it is best to clean the lesion thoroughly and aspirate the fluid with a syringe. The drained blister can then be covered with a bandage to prevent infection and further trauma.

Furuncles and Carbuncles

Furuncles (boils) usually develop from a previous staphylococcal folliculitis and frequently involve hair-bearing areas such as the face, scalp, axillae, and buttocks. The furuncles are usually red, tender nodules which rupture and discharge necrotic material. Carbuncles are more deeply situated than furuncles and drain at multiple points in the skin. They are often located on the posterior neck, back, and thighs. Small furuncles can usually be managed with moist heat. Larger furuncles and carbuncles should be carefully incised and drained when they become fluctuant. If the lesion is on the upper lip, nose, cheek, or forehead, or if there is an associated cellulitis or fever, systemic anti-staphylococcal antibiotics are indicated.

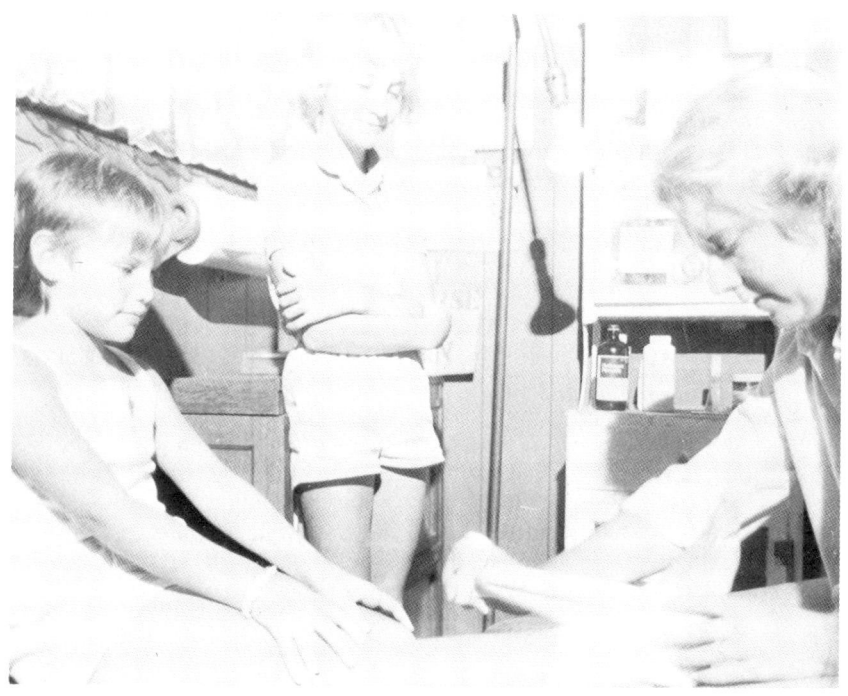

Impetigo

Impetigo is a contagious, superficial bacterial infection usually caused by the streptococcus with staphylococcus as a secondary invader; however, occasionally staphylococcus is the primary pathogen. The initial lesion of streptococcal impetigo is a thin-roofed pustule with surrounding erythema. Subsequently, the pustule breaks, leaving a red, eroded area which develops a golden-yellow crust. Impetigo due to a staphylococcus begins as a large flaccid bulla which then forms a superficial erosion with a thin crust. Lesions of impetigo may spread locally or become widespread.

Treatment of impetigo consists of topical and systemic therapy. Lesions should be soaked in warm tap water four times a day after which an antibacterial ointment (Polysporin®) should be applied. Systemic antibiotics are indicated for treatment of most cases of impetigo because this aids healing and decreases communicability. Streptococcal impetigo should be treated with intramuscular injection of benzathine penicillin (300,000-600,000 units for children; 1,200,000 units for adults) or oral penicillin (25,000-100,000 units/kg/day in four divided doses for 10 days). Erythromycin, 30-50 mg/kg/day in four divided doses in children or 250 mg four times a day for 10 days in adults may be used in patients allergic to penicillin. Staphylococcal impetigo should be treated with dicloxicillin (12.5 mg/kg/day in equally divided doses every six hours in children less than 40 kg, 125 mg every six hours in adults and children greater than 40 kg) or erythromycin (30 to 50 mg/kg/day in divided doses in children or 250 mg four times daily in adults) for 10 days. Food handlers should be relieved of their duties until skin lesions have cleared.

Urticaria

Urticaria is a common hypersensitivity reaction to a number of exogenous agents including drugs, food, food additives, inhalants, contactants, or parasitic infections. Uncommonly, urticaria may be a manifestation of internal diseases such as infections, collagen vascular diseases, and malignant tumors. In addition, urticaria may rarely be due to physical stimuli such as heat, cold, pressure, or light. The cause of the urticaria is determined in less than 10 percent of cases.

Clinically, urticarial wheals are erythematous, raised, edematous plaques usually with well-defined borders and surrounding erythema. Individual lesions range from several millimeters to several centimeters in size and persist for 8-18 hours. The lesions are usually very pruritic or burning in quality. History may occasionally reveal the cause of urticaria. If urticaria persists for more than six weeks, a complete medical evaluation should be done.

Therapy begins by removing the causative agent if that can be determined. Local measures include cool compresses and antipruritic lotions such as 1/4 percent menthol and 1 percent phenol in Lubriderm®. Systemic medications begin with antihistamines. Hydroxyzine (Atarax®) is among the most effective agents available. Dosage should begin at about 25 mg at bedtime and should be increased with divided doses during the day until the urticaria is controlled or until the medication is no longer tolerated. If this drug is not effective, other antihistamines, either singly or in combination, may be tried. Cyproheptadine hydrochloride (Periactin®) is frequently a helpful additon to the regimen. In acute, severe urticaria, particularly if there is potential airway obstruction, 0.1-0.5 ml (maximum) of subcutaneous epinephrine (1:1000) in addition to administration of antihistamines intramuscularly should be used. Systemic steroids are seldom needed in treating urticaria.

Verrucae

Verrucae, or warts, are common growths on the skin and are due to the human papilloma virus. Lesions are papular with a firm, thickened surface. Verrucae may involve any skin surface, but hands and feet are particularly prone.

Since warts are due to an infectious agent, they are auto-inoculable and contagious. The clinical course is benign and usually slowly progressive. Therefore, therapy is most often not justified in the camp setting. Plantar warts (warts on the soles) may be tender and small pads in the shoes may help redistribute weight and decrease irritation. Definitive therapy is best delayed until after the camp season is over.

Ringworm

Ringworm (dermatophyte) fungi cause superficial infections in man involving primarily epidermal keratin, hair, and nails. Poor nutrition, debilitating disease, contact with animals or humans and contaminated or infected soil, plus poor hygiene all contribute to the likelihood of acquiring the infection. Tinea capitis (ringworm of the scalp) and tinea corporis (ringworm of the body) are the most common dermatophyte infections seen in children. Fungal infections of the hands and nails are relatively infrequent in the camper age group.

Tinea capitis is very contagious and epidemics may occur. Organisms probably gain entrance through abraded skin. Ringworm of the scalp is usually asymptomatic; however, when significant edema and inflammation are present (kerion), the lesions may be painful. Physical findings include patchy hair loss, broken hairs, and scaling of the scalp. When kerion formation is present, the lesion is swollen, purulent, and tender.

Tinea corporis is usually asymptomatic or may be mildly pruritic. Typical lesions start as small macules and then gradually enlarge to form annular plaques with scaling borders and healing centers. Lesions are usually single but may be multiple.

Tinea cruris ("jock strap itch"), manuum (hands), and pedis ("athlete's foot") are usually exacerbated by friction, maceration, and summertime heat. Causative fungi can frequently be isolated from floors, bathing areas, shoes, and socks. The main symptom of tinea of the groin and feet is intense pruritus. The physical findings of tinea cruris are symmetrical, well-defined erythematous plaques in the groin and upper thighs. Tinea manuum and pedis commonly show interdigital scaling and may progress to significant palmar scaling and/or vesicular eruption.

Different species of dermatophyte fungi vary as to the site on the human host which they infect. Tinea capitis is most frequently due to *Trichophyton tonsaurans*, *Microsporum audouini*, or *Microsporum canis*. Tinea corporis is commonly due to *Trichophyton mentagrophytes*, *Trichophyton rubrum*, or *Epidermophyton floccosum*. Tinea manuum, pedis, and cruris are frequently caused by *Trichophyton mentagrophytes* and *Trichophyton rubrum*.

Diagnosis is established by (a) microscopic identification of fungi in skin scale, hair, or nails, or (b) culture. When obtaining a sample for microscopy, lesions should be gently scraped with a number 15 scalpel blade and the scale placed on a microscope slide. Scrapings should be covered with 10 percent potassium hydroxide (KOH) and then overlaid with a coverslip. The specimen should then be gently heated but not boiled for approximately 15 seconds. The slide is then blotted and examined for hyphae and spores. A species diagnosis cannot be made from skin scrapings. For culture, skin scale from the lesion should be placed on Sabouraud's agar with chloramphenicol and actidione (Mycosel). Cultures should be incubated at room temperature and examined at two to four weeks. Wood's light (ultraviolet light A, 320-400 nm) causes blue-green fluorescence of hairs infected with *Microsporum audouini* or *Microsporum canis*. However, tinea capitis due to *Trichophyton tonsaurans* and many other fungi do not fluoresce.

Treatment of ringworm infections differs depending on the anatomic location involved. Tinea capitis responds well to micronized griseofulvin orally in a dose of 5 mg per pound of body weight per day in divided doses. In general, treatment should continue for about two weeks after cultures become negative and lesions have clinically resolved, with a total treatment time usually lasting six to eight weeks. Topical anti-fungals are of no benefit when used in addition to griseofulvin, but good local hygiene is important. Tinea corporis, when localized, will usually respond to topical clotrimazole (Lotrimin®) or miconazole (Monistat Derm®) applied three times daily to affected areas until mycologic and clinical cure are achieved. If the tinea corporis is widespread or resistant, oral griseofulvin may also be needed. Tinea cruris or pedis can often be controlled with topical miconazole or clotrimazole, but systemic griseofulvin will sometimes be necessary for control. In the camp setting it is best to attempt control of the infection with topical and hygenic measures. Measures to decrease surface moisture such as thorough drying after bathing, absorbent cotton clothing, and nonocclusive footwear are also helpful when treating tinea cruris and pedis. Frequent laundering of towels and clothing may also hasten resolution of ringworm infections and prevent spread to others. If appropriately treated, patients with dermatophyte infections do not need to be isolated.

Insect Bites

Most reactions to insect bites, such as those caused by bees, hornets, yellow jackets, wasps, fleas, ants, and mosquitos, are due to acquired sensitivity to injected venom. Venom from Hymenoptera (bee and wasp) stings contains serotonin and kinins among other chemical agents, and hypersensitivity reactions to these compounds usually manifest as anaphylaxis. True toxic reactions (see below) to injected venom may also occur.

The usual reaction to a Hymenoptera sting in a non-allergic individual is local pain and pruritus. The reaction is manifested by a red area with a central punctum. Later a short-lived wheal may develop. If a non-allergic individual is stung by multiple insects, then true toxic reactions may take place such as intense pain at the site of the bites and in addition, nausea, vomiting, headache, fever, and vertigo. The cutaneous features may be in the form of edema and redness. Hymenoptera stings in allergic individuals may result in an anaphylactic reaction with urticaria, abdominal cramping, bronchospasm, laryngeal edema, and shock.

Reactions to ant stings are often caused by harvester or fire ants. The usual reaction is intense burning, with a wheal topped by two hemorrhagic puncta. These lesions evolve into vesiculo-pustules which then form crusts, followed by possible scar formation. The allergic reaction to mosquito bites produces intense pruritus. The initial lesion is a wheal followed in several hours by a papule. Reactions to flies, such as the blackfly, produce pruritic nodular or nodulovesicular lesions. Flea bites usually produce urticarial papules with a central punctum.

When insects bite, they should be flicked off the skin in order to remove the venom sac. Squeezing the insect may inject venom into the bite. If the stinger is not removed, it should be gently extracted with tweezers or a clean blade. Cold compresses may decrease absorption of the venom and help to decrease the inflammatory response. Lotions containing 1/4 percent menthol and 1/2 percent phenol may be soothing, and topical corticosteroids may decrease inflammation. Antihistamines are useful for the control of pruritus.

Systemic allergic reactions manifesting as mild anaphylaxis should be treated with 0.01 ml/kg epinephrine HCl (1:1000) given subcutaneously. If the reaction is more severe, the epinephrine may be administered intramuscularly. Administration of an antihistamine such as chlorpheniramine (Chlor-trimeton®), 5-10 mg every six hours, or diphenhydramine (Benadryl®), 25-50 mg every six hours (depending on the child's size) either orally or intramuscularly may also be helpful. For laryngeal edema, epinephrine is again the treatment of choice and hydrocortisone 100 mg every six hours intravenously is indicated. If the airway is seriously compromised, either tracheostomy or endotracheal intubation should be performed. Theophylline and hydrocortisone should be administered for bronchoconstriction. Pressor agents are indicated for severe hypotension. Good medical monitoring and support are needed for severe reactions. If immunizations are not up to date, all patients with serious bites should receive tetanus prophylaxis. Campers who need this type of care should be transferred to the nearest hospital.

Patients with known sensitivity to Hymenoptera stings should carry a kit which contains a syringe loaded with epinephrine, tourniquet, and antihistamine tablets. Preventive measures include wearing protective clothing that is not brightly colored. Perfumes and scents may attract insects and should be avoided. Insect repellents containing diethyltoluamide are effective against wasps and bees. It may be necessary to apply the repellent liberally every hour, depending on the density of the insects. Desensitization procedures are effective in reducing the sensitivity of severely allergic individuals. Immunotherapy should be strongly considered in those who have had severe local or systemic reactions and should be completed before arriving at camp.

Cercariae Dermatitis (Swimmer's Itch)

Cercariae are encountered along the lake districts of the northern United States and along both fresh and salt water areas along the east and west coasts. The cercariae are blood flukes of aquatic birds or domestic animals. The cercariae invade the human epidermis and produce an intensive itching and the appearance of an erythematous maculopapular rash. A shower with the use of copious amounts of soap after swimming in contaminated water may help. Treatment consists of Lubriderm® cream containing 1 percent phenol applied several times a day locally and antihistamines by mouth. If large areas of the body are affected, a Lubriderm® bath oil might be used for tub baths. The camp director should report such contamination to the local public health authorities who may help in the treatment of the swimming area.

References

Arndt, K. *Manual of Dermatologic Therapeutics.* Boston. Little, Brown and Company, 1978.
Fitzpatrick, T.B., Eisen, A.Z., Wolff, K., Freedberg, I. M., Austen, K. F. *Dermatology in General Medicine.* New York. McGraw-Hill Book Company, 1979.

Chapter IX

ALLERGIC DISORDERS

by Donald B. Strominger*
Clinical Professor of Pediatrics
Department of Pediatrics
Washington University School of Medicine

Allergic disorders are a common health problem in children, causing more school absences than any other condition. It is understandable that such children will arrive at summer camp with a variety of medications and injections with instructions from their parents ranging from which foods are forbidden to the amount of daily sun exposure tolerated. Fortunately, most of the disorders are more of an inconvenience than life-threatening.

Immunotherapy

A number of campers may be on an immunotherapy program that requires regular injections of allergens. Each child will have his own vial of extract with special instructions. In most cases, a multiple-dose vial will be used, but occasionally single-dose vials will be sent. The injections should be given subcutaneously in the lateral aspect of the left arm (if the child is right-handed), midway between the shoulder and elbow. In the event of a systemic reaction, a tourniquet should be applied above the injection site and approximately 0.1 ml of 1:1000 aqueous epinephrine injected into and around the immunotherapy site. Aqueous epinephrine should be injected into the opposite arm (subcutaneously, if no emergency; intramuscularly with massage if symptoms are alarming). Further supportive measures may be necessary, but this is not likely. Large local reactions are of no concern unless they last more than 12 hours or if the entire extremity becomes swollen. If this happens, the next injection of the allergen should be cut to one-third the dose that elicited the "local" reaction.

Allergic Rhinitis and Conjunctivitis

The patient with allergic rhinitis may have seasonal or perennial symptoms, depending on the offending antigens. There is usually a history of an itching, watery nose or eyes with rubbing or an "allergic salute." The nasal mucous membranes are swollen and have a bluish tinge. The conjunctivae may be reddened and may have a cobblestone appearance. The eyelids may swell. Occasionally, there will be so much edema and swelling that the eustachian tubes will be blocked, causing either hearing loss

---

*Deceased 1983.

or fluid accumulation in the middle ear with pain and secondary infection.
Treatment of this annoying disorder should consist of an antihistamine and either Naphcon® or Vasocon® eye drops when necessary.

Asthma

It is possible that a young child will have his first asthmatic attack at camp. Therefore, a preceding history may not be available. The more primitive the camp, the higher is the concentration of mold. The more rural the camp is, the higher the concentration of pollens. A good guide to follow is that plants pollinate from sunup, reaching a peak at about 8:00 or 9:00 a.m., and are greatly decreased by noon. Rain will help cleanse the air of pollens. Molds sporulate immediately after sunset and peak in the early evening and nighttime hours. Rain and dampness increase the level of molds.

An asthmatic attack may be characterized by a slow insidious onset with upper respiratory symptoms, which may progress to a cough or wheeze. If the exposure is sudden, an acute attack may occur. Symptoms may vary from a chronic deep cough to a frank wheeze and/or shortness of breath. The patient may have a vague feeling of inability to catch his breath. Mortality from asthma does not occur suddenly, but rather from progressive, prolonged disease (*status asthmaticus*). In any severe attack, a pneumomediastinum may occur with air dissecting into the neck. This is not dangerous but is an indication of the severity of the attack. Consequently, medications may be given reasonably and without panic.

The following is a suggested therapeutic approach for a child having an asthmatic attack:

1. Air conditioning and isolation in a quiet room may abort or relieve an attack.
2. Remove the offending antigen when possible.
3. Force clear liquids to keep the thick mucus from inspissating in the airway.
4. Administer aqueous epinephrine (1:1000) 0.01 ml/kg (maximum 0.4 ml) subcutaneously which may be repeated in 15-30 minutes for a maximum of three doses.
5. Start theophylline, 5 mg/kg/dose every 4-6 hours (maintain on long-acting preparations at 10 mg/kg twice a day).
6. Aerosol of Alupent® every two hours may be as effective as repeated injections of epinephrine (0.3 ml Alupent in 2 ml of normal saline and inhaled with the aid of a nasal nebulizer).
7. Alupent®, 10 mg (under 60 lbs.) or 20 mg (over 60 lbs.) by mouth three to four times a day.
8. Increase steroids for patients who are already on them or give a short course of 10 mg prednisone three times a day, then 10 mg twice daily for three days, and 10 mg daily for three days if the attack is severe.

It should be emphasized that if the camper does not respond to therapy in 24 hours, the camper should be transferred to the nearest local hospital for further treatment after the parents are notified about their child's progress.

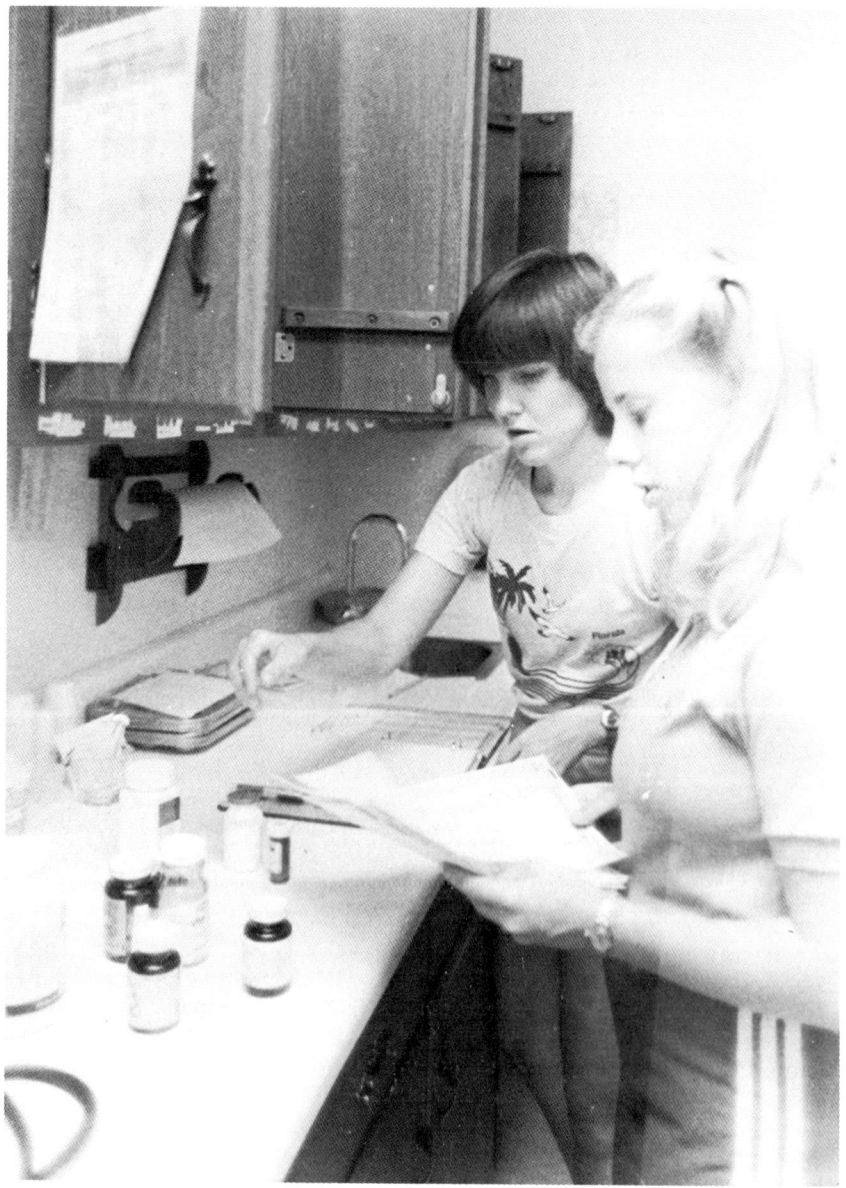

Chapter X

EYE INJURIES AND INFECTIONS

If a camper sustains an injury to his eye by a blow or a ball he should have cool compresses applied, and if the discomfort disappears in one to two hours, the injury is probably not serious. If complaints persist for 24 hours, the camper should be examined by the camp physician and then if indicated, referred to an ophthalmologist for an opinion.

It should be emphasized that even minor injuries to the eye deserve the utmost care and consideration. Small abrasions and superficial foreign bodies will cause acute pain and prompt the camper to seek aid.

Ecchymosis and edema are signs of injury to the eyelids. Ecchymosis (black eye) is usually not serious if the eyeball is not involved. A camper with such a condition should be examined daily for evidence of possible complications.

Lacerations of the eyelid are generally more extensive than they appear externally. A small wound on the skin surface may not reflect the extent of the laceration of the tarsus. Prompt and complete examination by an expert ophthalmologist is therefore indicated.

Foreign Bodies in the Eye

Usually a camper will know when a foreign body has lodged in his eye. Sudden onset of pain with tearing and congestion of the conjunctivae is highly suggestive of a foreign body on the cornea or conjunctivae. Foreign bodies may be located by examination with a condensed light and a magnifying glass.

If the foreign body is on the lower lid, this can be removed by the nurse with an applicator made of a tuft of cotton wound tightly upon a toothpick and moistened with water. If there is no visible foreign body in the eye, the foreign body may have lodged on the upper lid, and the nurse may remove this by everting the upper lid. This is easily done by grasping the eyelashes of the temporal portion of the upper lid. Have the patient look down. Place the thumb or an applicator on the outer margin of the lid. With the lid pulled down and slightly outwards, the hand holding the lashes suddenly everts the lid outward on the indenting instrument or finger. If the foreign body is seen, this can be removed as explained above. If the foreign body is not seen, the patient should be seen by the physician. He/she should first have the camper wash his eye gently in a full glass of water by opening and closing his eyelids while the eye is submerged. Next, a fluorescin strip should be placed inside the lower lid of the eye for several seconds. This will stain an abrasion. Defects on the cornea stain green and those on the conjunctivae stain yellow. Foreign bodies on the cornea may best be seen with an ophthalmoscope. Irregularities upon the surface may show the location of the foreign body. Foreign bodies should be removed with an instrument which is not sharp enough to penetrate the globe and which will lift rather than dig out the foreign body. Sometimes a foreign body can be flushed out with normal saline. Two percent homatropine and a 1/4 percent zinc sulfate should be instilled, and a sterile pad should be placed over the eye. If a foreign body is suspected and none found, the patient should be referred to an ophthalmologist for evaluation.

It is not advisable to use a moist cotton swab to remove a corneal foreign body, because the cotton may be sufficiently abrasive to remove a considerable amount of corneal epithelium. Metallic corneal foreign bodies usually cause rust stains. It is advisable to have an ophthalmologist remove the rust stains. Occasionally, multiple foreign bodies will be seen in the cornea. This may occur following the backfire of a gun or by the spontaneous explosion of a bicycle tire.

Usually these foreign bodies extrude themselves, but it is imperative that the camper be followed by an ophthalmologist. If the physician is not experienced at removing foreign bodies from the eye, he should not atempt it for the first time in a camp situation. It might be well to mention the serious nature of lime burns, in view of the use of lime on tennis courts, in latrines, etc. Copious irrigation with water is necessary to remove free-floating particles from the eye. All lime particles should be removed manually from the conjunctivae as soon as possible.

Hemorrhages

Blood present over or on the surface of the sclera of the eye may occur spontaneously or following trauma. This subconjunctival hemorrhage may concentrate around the periphery of the cornea. The blood is absorbed over several days. Blood present in front of the pupil of the eye (hyphema) is a serious problem and consultation by an ophthalmologist is necessary. All eye injuries should be seen by the camp physician for evaluation. In case of an eye injury, it is wise to have the camper seen by an ophthalmologist after first aid is administered by the camp physician.

Hordeolum (Sty)

Relatively few infections of the eyes are seen at camp. Occasionally a camper may be seen with an hordeolum or sty. This is an infection of the follicle of an eyelash and is usually caused by the staphylococcus. The infection produces redness, swelling, pain, tenderness, and sometimes preauricular adenopathy. Sties tend to occur in series. Incision should not be done, but pulling the affected cilium (lash) often results in drainage. Warm compresses will facilitate drainage.

Chalazion

This is an inflammation of the Meibomian gland resulting in a tumor-like swelling of the border of the eyelid. These are frequently mistaken for a sty. Treatment consists of antimicrobial ophthalmic drops (4 percent Gantrisin Solution) and warm local compresses to the eye several times daily. Failure of response to therapy in several days requires referral to an ophthalmologist.

Bacterial Conjunctivitis (Pink Eye)

Upon occasion, an outbreak of "pink eye" may occur in camp. This is an acute bacterial conjunctivitis and deserves comment because it is contagious and has the potential of becoming an epidemic. There are other infections and inflammations of the eye with which this may be confused.

"Pink eye" is a disease characterized by lacrimation, irritation, discharge, and vascular injection of the bulbar and palpebral conjunctivae. The lids may be edematous, and the camper will complain of a scratchy sensation. The patient usually recovers in four to five days.

The most frequent etiologic agents are the staphylococcus, pneumococcus, and streptococcus. Other organisms incriminated are *Haemophilus aegyptius, Haemophilus influenzae,* and *Moraxella lacunatas.*

The disease is transmitted by contact with infected individuals through contaminated hands, towels, handkerchiefs, etc. The incubation period is two to three days.

The infected individual and the counselor should be instructed about personal hygiene and about the mode of spread of the infection. The camper should be restricted from swimming. Dark sunglasses will make the camper more comfortable. Cold compresses are sometimes helpful. Cleaning the eye free of purulent secretions three to four times a day and the installation of antimicrobial ophthalmic drops during the daytime and ointments at night, such as sulfacetamide, bacitracin, and/or Polymyxin® are effective. Steroid therapy should be avoided.

A number of inflammatory or infectious conditions may be confused with "pink eye," and these are covered briefly in the following discussions.

Keratoconjunctivitis

This is an acute infection of the eyes which is usually bilateral. It may be preceded by an upper respiratory infection. The onset is marked by fever, headache, edema of the lids, scleral injection, follicular hypertrophy of the palpebral conjunctivae, enlargement and tenderness of the preauricular lymph nodes, and a watery conjunctival discharge. Sometimes this is followed by pinpoint corneal opacities which clear spontaneously.

The etiologic agent is felt to be a virus, and the diagnosis is suspected if the smears made of conjunctival scrapings show mononuclear cells.

The transmission of the disease is by direct contact with infected individuals or articles soiled by the infected individual. The incubation period is approximately five to seven days. The camper should be restricted from swimming, and he and his counselor should be instructed about the importance of personal hygiene and the mode of spread of the infection. Cold compresses help in making the camper more comfortable, and antibiotics should be given if there is evidence of secondary bacterial infection.

Inclusion Blennorrhea

Acute inclusion conjunctivitis may be a viral or chlamydial infection and inclusions are much harder to find in conjunctival scrapings from older children and adults. These may occur as a result of contamination of swimming pools. This infection requires both topical and systemic sulfonamide therapy. Tetracycline may be used in children over eight years of age.

Vernal Conjunctivitis

This is an allergic disturbance which tends to occur in warm weather and disappears with the onset of winter. Symptoms include lacrimation, intense itching, and photophobia. In the palpebral form there are hard, flattened papillae on the upper palpebral conjunctiva, producing a cobblestone appearance, and a bluish-white color of the upper and lower palpebral conjunctivae as though covered with a thin layer of milk. In the bulbar form, the conjunctiva adjacent to the limbus presents gelatinous elevations. The conjunctiva is congested and has a stringy mucoid secretion which contains eosinophils.

The symptoms can be relieved by irrigation with a normal saline solution; a 1:3000 epinephrine solution and cold compresses will be helpful. Topical antihistamines may be helpful. Topical steroids are sometimes recommended, but this should be decided by an ophthalmologist, because bacterial infection may be mistaken for vernal conjunctivitis by the inexperienced physician.

Blepharitis

This is an inflammation which principally involves the margins of the eyelids and the skin around the base of the cilia. Redness, scales, crusts, and ulcerations may be present. The lashes are often matted by cellular debris and exudates. Sometimes the lashes may be lost and trichiasis may result. Seborrhea is a common cause. This may occur alone or be complicated by secondary infection. Treatment of the seborrhea of the scalp and brows is essential to the clearing of the marginal blepharitis. Staphylococcal infections of the glands of the skin and hair follicles and of the Meibomian glands are common. Soap and water cleansing may be helpful. Non-stinging baby shampoos have been found helpful in the treatment of the lashes.

A few general remarks need to be made.

1. Most forms of bacterial conjunctivitis respond to antibiotic ophthalmic drops.
2. Homatropine, 2 percent, is better to use following removal of a corneal foreign body because the effect of atropine solutions may last up to two weeks.
3. In the event of an injury to the eye, a letter should be sent to the parents about the accident, treatment, etc.

Chapter XI

BITES BY SNAKES, ANIMALS, AND SPIDERS

Bites by Snakes

It is estimated that there are approximately 8,000 persons bitten by venomous snakes in the United States each year. Nine to 14 of these people die from the bite. Epidemiological studies show that 30 percent were in persons under 15 years of age, 25 percent in the 15-20 year age group and another 33 percent among those 20-30 years old. The bites were on one of the extremities in 98 percent (57 percent lower, 41 percent upper), with only 2 percent occurring on the face and trunk. The real danger from snakebite is tissue destruction and residual dysfunction of a finger, hand, arm, or leg.

The most common poisonous snakes in this country belong to the subfamily Crotalinae or "pit vipers," and include the rattlesnake, cottonmouth, and copperhead. The Crotalinae are called "pit vipers" because of the depression that is located midway between the eye and nostril. The "pit" is thought to function as a radiant energy detector. The venom is secreted by a pair of glands on either side of the head. The venom is thought to initiate digestion of the body of the prey through enzyme action. The glands are connected to hollow fangs which are attached to the maxilla and fold inward when the mouth is shut. During a strike the fangs unfold and are long enough to reach muscle tissue.

The other poisonous snake in the United States is the coral snake. The bite of a coral snake is extremely rare. The venom attacks the nervous system, especially the part which controls the muscles and respiration. Systemic symptoms and signs include drowsiness, weakness, fasciculation and tremors of the tongue, difficulty in swallowing, increased salivation, nausea, and vomiting. Paresis of extraocular muscles, pinpoint pupils, and dyspnea have been reported. Convulsions, hypotension, and paralysis of limbs and respirations may also occur. Death results from cardiac and respiratory failure. Treatment with specific antivenin is recommended.

The composition of venom and pharmacologic aspects are imperfectly understood. Venoms have a chemically complex structure and have been demonstrated to contain at least 26 enzymes, although no single venom contains all of these. These include protease, collagenase, hyaluronidase, phospholipase, phosphodiesterase, acetylcholinesterase, polypeptides, and procoagulant and anticoagulant activities. The activity of the venom results in digestion and necrosis of tissue, hemorrhage and dissolution of red blood cells, endothelium, and lymphatics resulting in those changes seen locally at the site of envenomation.

The toxic effects of the venom are classified as (a) primary—which is usually an irreversible, destructive effect upon tissues and organs, and (b) secondary—the components of the venom promote the release of substances from the tissues such as histamine, bradykinin, and unsaturated fatty acids which act primarily upon smooth muscle; lysolecithin, which alters cell permeability; and adenyl compounds, which act on the conduction mechanism of the heart.

Neurotoxic and hematoxic actions are common to most, if not all, snake venoms. The neurotoxic actions of venoms are exerted on the myoneural junction and the central nervous system.

The cardiovascular actions affect the myocardium and the conduction mechanism of the heart; smooth and skeletal muscle are also affected. The venom may produce vasoconstriction or vasodilation of blood vessels. There is also a change in permeability and disintegration of smaller vessels and an alteration of the blood-clotting mechanism.

Snake envenomization is always potentially serious. Bites on the face are always more serious than bites upon the extremities. The amount of venom injected in relation to the size of the victim has an important bearing upon the prognosis.

Death from snakebite usually does not occur for several hours or days. The outcome is determined by the time between the bite and the institution of treatment and whether an adequate amount of antivenin was given. Those who survive without rapid, adequate treatment may be left with deep scars, contractures, and paresthesia or an amputation as permanent sequelae.

Most bites result from carelessness and failure to follow certain precautions in the field, which are as follows:

1. Rubber or leather knee-high boots should be worn in the field.
2. Watch where you put your hands when climbing.
3. Don't thrust your hands or feet under rock ledges, logs, or stumps.
4. Use long poles to overturn logs or rocks.
5. Stay on paths or trails and watch where you walk.
6. Handle any dead snake with care. Reflex action may last for a long time, and supposedly dead copperheads and rattlesnakes have been known to bite.
7. Never leave the group in an area where snakes are prevalent.

The fangs of a poisonous snake produce two distinct punctures. There may also be a circular row of minute wounds from the small teeth of the lower jaw as both venomous and nonvenomous snakes have small teeth. The bite of a nonvenomous snake causes marks similar to scratches.

After a venomous snakebite there is almost instantaneous swelling and edema of the skin at the site of the injury with varying degrees of local pain. Nausea and vomiting follow very shortly thereafter. The severity of the reaction is governed by the amount of venom which is introduced. The victim may become faint and dizzy. He may break out in a cold sweat. The blood pressure may fall and the pulse may become fast and feeble. Muscular tremors, numbness, lethargy, and paralysis may develop, and convulsions may be seen, especially in children.

The camp director should plan upon indoctrination of his counseling staff in the prevention and treatment of snakebite in the field in a camp which is located in an area where snakes are prevalent. If a camper is bitten by a poisonous snake, he should be stretched out on the ground and kept warm and at rest. The area of the bite should be cleansed with soap and water. An immediate incision should be made at the site of the bite, and the venom suctioned either by a suction cup or by mouth. This should be carried out for 30 to 60 minutes (the venom is destroyed if swallowed). The incision should be no more than one centimeter in length and no deeper than three millimeters. This procedure should be done within 15 minutes following the bite if it is to be of value and cruciate incisions are not necessary. This maneuver may be of value in the field. The use of a tourniquet above the bite is of questionable value and may injure the tissue if it is applied too tightly. The use of cool, wet applications may be of help in making the camper more comfortable and may help reduce the degree of swelling.

The counselor should call the Health Supervisor at camp and inform him that the camper has been bitten by a snake. The Health Supervisor should be well informed about the immediate treatment of snakebite and plan to transfer the victim to a hospital after emergency treatment has been given.

When the camper arrives, he should be put at rest and the injured extremity should be immobilized. The site of the bite should be cleansed with soap and water. Most experts do not recommend cooling of the extremity. Aspirin, acetaminophen, or codeine are sufficient to control pain in most cases. Meperidine may be necessary, but may provoke more vomiting in many cases. In the severely poisoned patient, it may be advisable to administer an intravenous infusion of 5 percent glucose or Ringer's lactate solution to maintain blood pressure. Tetanus toxoid or tetanus immune globulin (human) should be given as in any other puncture wound, and a broad-spectrum antibiotic is indicated. The wound should not be cauterized.

Antivenin should be given only if the bite has been inflicted by a large snake or if the bite is on the face of the camper and if he is more than 20-30 minutes from medical care. The antivenin should be administered by a physician when possible. The reason for this is that the camper may be allergic to the horse serum and may have an allergic reaction severe enough to cause death.

Antihistamines, steroids, heparin, and ethylene diamine tetracetate (EDTA) have no place in the acute treatment of snakebite. Antihistamines and steroids do have a place in the control of antivenin hypersensitivity or serum reactions.

The most important therapeutic step is the administration of antivenin. Antivenin (Crotalinae) Polyalent was developed by the Wyeth Laboratories and is prepared from hyperimmune horse serum. It contains protective substances against the venoms of the Crotalinae (pit vipers). The dried antiserum in vials is readily soluble in water. It has been shown that potency persists for three to five years in the dried state in intact vials. Anitvenin may be carried in the field at temperatures encountered in the open without loss of potency. Refrigeration is recommended for prolonged storage. Similarly, Wyeth Laboratories have an antivenin for coral snakes (Antivenin Micrurus fulvius).

If the patient is allergic to horse serum, the physician must weigh the risk of the allergic reaction against the potential danger of envenomization. In severe envenomization, the risk of administering the serum is warranted even in an allergic patient if the serum is administered properly.

The amount of antivenin administered depends on many factors, the most important being the severity and rapidity of progression of the signs and symptoms. The girth and circumference of the finger, toe, hand, or foot and two or more proximal sites should be marked and then measured. These measurements can be repeated every 15 to 30 minutes and serve as an index of progression and guideline for antivenin therapy.

In most snake bites, the administration of three to five vials of antivenin intravenously is usually sufficient. The antivenin is mixed with the diluent in the vial and transferred to a 5 percent glucose in Ringer's lactate solution at a 1:10 dilution and administered in one to two hours. Epinephrine (1:1000) and Benadryl® should be kept on hand in the event of a serum reaction.

In snake bites where edema has involved the hand or foot, and if within 30 minutes it is progressing and mild cyanosis or ecchymosis of the area is present and is associated with nausea or weakness; peripheral paresthesia; tingling of the scalp, finger, or toe; or hypotension, six to ten vials of antivenin should be given. Some physicians inject one-third of a vial of antivenin subcutaneously in the area of the bite, but antivenin should never be injected into a finger or toe. The antivenin is most effective if given within four hours of the bite.

In coral snake bites (rare in the United States), three to five vials of antivenin (Mircrurus fulvius) should be given intravenously within the first several hours following the bite if symptoms and signs develop.

Sensitivity Testing for Serum Reaction

Never inject a serum or perform a skin test unless a syringe containing 1 ml of 1:1000 epinephrine is within immediate reach.

It should be stressed that when a camper or one of the camp personnel is very sensitive to horse serum, he should be transferred to a hospital where the administration of the antiserum can be carried out with greater safety.

An intracutaneous skin test, preceded by a scratch or eye test, should always be done before injecting any animal serum, whether or not the patient has had the serum previously. A scratch test is performed by applying a drop of 1:100 saline dilution of the serum to the site of a superficial scratch and observing it for 30 minutes. A positive reaction consists of erythema or wheal formation.

An eye test is performed by instilling a drop of 1:10 saline dilution of serum in one eye and a drop of physiologic saline solution in the other eye to serve as a control. A positive reaction consists of lacrimation and conjunctivitis appearing in 10 to 30 minutes.

If the scratch test or eye test is negative, an intradermal test is performed by injecting 0.1 ml of a 1:100 saline dilution. The reaction is read after 10 to 30 minutes and is positive if a wheal appears. In persons with a history of allergy, the dose is reduced to 0.05 ml of a 1:1000 dilution, intradermally.

Skin and eye tests can indicate the probability of sensitivity. However, a negative skin or eye test is not an absolute guarantee of absence of sensitivity. Therefore, either a specific history of allergy to or a positive skin or eye test with horse serum is sufficient reason for special caution. A positive history of sensitivity to horse dander is an indication for extreme caution.

If the history and sensitivity tests are negative, the indicated dose of serum may be given intramuscularly.

If the skin test is positive or there is a history of allergy in a person who needs serum therapy, 1 ml of 1:10 dilution of the serum in physiologic saline may be administered subcutaneously and given low enough in one of the extremities so that a tourniquet could be placed above the site of the injection if a severe reaction should occur. The patient should be watched for one-half hour. *Epinephrine should be at hand.*

If no reaction appears, 1 ml of undiluted serum should be given subcutaneously and the patient should be observed for another half hour. If there still is no reaction, proceed as indicated above. If a reaction occurs, a procedure commonly called "desensitization" is undertaken, but it is dangerous to assume that any significant desensitization occurs. It is more likely that this procedure merely results in establishing the tolerance level of the patient. A suggested procedure is as follows:

Inject the following doses every 15 minutes, if no reaction occurs:

1. 0.5 ml of 1:20 dilution, subcutaneously
2. 0.1 ml of 1:10 dilution, subcutaneously
3. 0.3 ml of 1:10 dilution, subcutaneously
4. 0.1 ml of undiluted serum, subcutaneously
5. 0.2 ml of undiluted serum, subcutaneously
6. 0.5 ml of undiluted serum, subcutaneously
7. inject remaining therapeutic dose intramuscularly

Three types of reactions may occur: an immediate anaphylactic reaction, serum sickness, or an acute febrile episode.

Acute anaphylactic reactions consist of urticaria, dyspnea, cyanosis, shock, and unconsciousness that occurs seconds to minutes after an injection. These are critical emergencies.

The treatment of an anaphylactic reaction is as follows: epinephrine 1:1000 (0.01 ml/kg) is given immediately either subcutaneously or intramuscularly. If there is not immediate improvement, epinephrine 1:1000 at a dose of 0.01 ml/kg, maximum dose of 0.5 ml, is given intravenously. The 1:1000 epinephrine must be diluted 1:10 in physiologic saline and injected slowly. An intravenous infusion of physiologic saline is started immediately. Epinephrine may be repeated in 5 to 15 minutes if the response is not satisfactory. Vasopressors and positive pressure oxygen are helpful. For severe urticaria or edema, particularly edema of the larynx, intramuscular injection of diphenhydramine (Benedryl®) 2 mg/kg or 5 mg/kg/24 hr (25-50 mg q4h) orally is indicated. Hydrocortisone 100-200 mg intravenously may be helpful. If serum therapy must be resumed, the camper should be transferred to a nearby hospital.

Serum sickness reactions consist of rash, urticaria, arthritis, adenopathy, and fever occurring hours or days after injection. Serum sickness occurs more frequently in persons who have previously received horse serum injections or received large doses of serum. The reaction may appear within a few hours to several days after the first injection. Serum sickness can be alleviated by salicylates, antihistamines, or corticosteroids.

Febrile reactions after animal serum injections are usually mild. Mild febrile reactions may be treated with salicylates and the usual symptomatic treatment of a fever. However, severe febrile reactions may cause death as a result of hyperpyrexia. Severe febrile reactions should be treated with salicylates or acetaminophen and tepid sponge baths to reduce the temperature, and the camper should be transferred to a hospital.

The local reactions may be of two types: (a) the local delayed serum reaction which may appear in one to twenty-four hours is manifested by progressive edema, erythema, and itching of the skin-tested area or the entire forearm; and (b) the Arthus phenomenon may occur at the site of the injection and results from repeated injections of antiserum at short intervals of less than 30 days. Local necrosis of the tissue develops at the site.

Any camper requiring intravenous antiserum (such as snake antivenin) should be transferred to a hospital.

Bites by Animals

Animal bites may cause severe infection—especially human bites. Bites on the face are especially dangerous. Lacerations and deep puncture wounds require energetic cleansing with soap and water, debridement, and primary closure. If the wound involves the face and is extensive or if there is the question of a severed tendon, it is wise to seek consultant help and have the repair done in a hospital. Cauterization should never be done, because this will increase the degree of injury. Protection against tetanus and prophylactic antibiotic therapy with penicillin and an antistaphylococcal drug are indicated.

In the case of an animal bite, antitetanus prophylaxis is given when indicated, but the chief concern of the camp physician is the question of antirabies treatment. It may be worthwhile to discuss the disease and its prevention and give the recommendations of the Advisory Committee for Immunization Practices for specific postexposure treatment *(Tables VI and VII).*

Rabies is invariably fatal because of an acute encephalitis in man which begins with headache, fever, and malaise and progresses to paresis and paralysis. When an attempt is made to drink, there is spasm of the muscles of swallowing. Delirium and convulsions follow, ending in death from respiratory paralysis. Verification of the diagnosis in man depends upon the demonstration of Negri bodies in the nerve cells of the brain or upon mouse inoculation of spinal fluid, throat and saliva specimens, or suspension of tissues obtained at autopsy.

The etiologic agent is the virus of rabies, and the source is the saliva of rabid animals such as the dog, fox, coyote, wolf, cat, skunk, raccoon, and opossum. Rabies is also carried by insectivorous bats producing no apparent disease in the bat.

The mode of transmission is by the bite of a rabid animal. On rare occasions, the disease may develop after aerosalization of the virus in the laboratory.

The incubation period is three to eight weeks and depends upon the extent of the laceration and the site of the wound in relation to the richness of the nerve supply and the length of the nerve path to the brain. The period of communicability in the dog is three to five days before the onset of clinical symptoms as well as throughout the course of the diesease.

Rabies is primarily a disease of animals and, fortunately, uncommon in man. Natural immunity in man is unknown. Prophylactic antirabies treatment of infected humans may prevent the disease if begun soon after injury.

Management of the biting animal when it is a healthy domestic dog or cat includes confinement and observation for ten days and evaluation by a veterinarian at the first signs of illness. If signs suggestive of rabies develop, the animal should be humanely killed without damage to the head. Its head should then be removed and shipped, under refrigeration, for examination by the local or state health department. Any stray or unwanted dog or cat that has bitten a person should be killed immediately and the head submitted for examination as described above for rabies examination.

Any wild animal that bites or scratches a person shall be killed at once (without damage to the head), and the brain examined for evidence of rabies. This incident should also be reported to local or state health authorities.

Table VI
Rabies Postexposure Prophylaxis Guide—1980

The following recommendations are only a guide. In applying them, take into account the animal species involved, the circumstances of the bite or other exposure, the vaccination status of the animal, and presence of rabies in the region. Local or state public health officials should be consulted if questions arise about the need for rabies prophylaxis.

	Animal Species	Condition of Animal at Time of Attack	Treatment of Exposed Person (1)
DOMESTIC	dog and cat	healthy and available for 10 days of observation	none, unless animal develops rabies (2)
		rabid or suspected rabid	RIG (3) and HDCV (4)
		unknown (escaped)	consult public health officials. If treatment is indicated, give RIG (3) and HDCV (4)
WILD	skunk, bat, fox, coyote, raccoon, bobcat, and other carnivores	regard as rabid unless proven negative by laboratory tests (5)	RIG (3) and HDCV (4)
OTHER	livestock, rodents, and lagomorphs (rabbits and hares)	Consider individually. Local and state public health officials should be consulted on questions about the need for rabies prophylaxis. Bites of squirrels, hamsters, guinea pigs, gerbils, chipmunks, rats, mice, other rodents, rabbits, and hares almost never call for antirabies prophylaxis.	

(1) All bites and wounds should be thoroughly cleansed with soap and water immediately. If antirabies treatment is indicated, both rabies immune globulin (RIG) and human diploid cell rabies vaccine (HDCV) should be given as soon as possible, regardless of the interval from exposure.

(2) During the usual holding period of 10 days, begin treatment with RIG and vaccine (preferably with HDCV) at first sign of rabies in a dog or cat that has bitten someone. The symptomatic animal should be killed immediately and tested.

(3) If RIG is not available, use antirabies serum, equine (ARS). Do not use more than the recommended dosage.

(4) If HDCV is not available, use duck embryo vaccine (DEV). Local reactions to vaccines are common and do not contraindicate continuing treatment. Discontinue vaccine if fluorescent-antibody (FA) tests of the animal are negative.

(5) The animal should be killed and tested as soon as possible. Holding for observation is not recommended.

Morbidity and Mortality Weekly Report. Center for Disease Control. 29: 279, June 13, 1980.

Table VII
Rabies Postexposure Immunization Schedule*

Postexposure rabies prophylaxis for persons exposed to rabies consists of the immediate, thorough cleansing of all wounds with soap and water, administration of rabies immune globulin (RIG) or, if RIG is not available, antirabies serum, equine (ARS), and the initiation of either HDCV or DEV, according to the following schedule. (3)

Rabies Vaccine	No. of 1 ml Doses	Route of Administration	Intervals Between Doses	If No Antibody Response to Primary Series, Give: (1)
HDCV	5 (4)	Intramuscular	Doses to be given on days 0, 3, 7, 14, and 28 (2)	An additional booster dose (2)
DEV	23	Subcutaneous	21 daily doses followed by a booster on day 31 and another on day 41 (2) or 2 daily doses in the first 7 days, followed by 7 daily doses. Then 1 booster on day 24, and another on day 34 (2)	3 doses of HDCV at weekly intervals (2)

(1) If no antibody response is documented after the recommended additional booster dose(s), consult the state health department or CDC.
(2) Serum for rabies antibody testing should be collected 2-3 weeks after the last dose.
(3) The postexposure regimen is greatly modified for someone with previously demonstrated rabies antibody. (See text for details.)
(4) The World Health Organization recommends a 6th dose 90 days after the first dose.

*Morbidity and Mortality Weekly Report. Center for Disease Control. 29: 280, June 13, 1980

Local and state public health officials should be consulted if questions arise about the need for rabies prophylaxis. Rabies immune globulin (RIG) or antirabies serum, equine (ARS) are administered only once, at the beginning of antirabies prophylaxis. The recommended dose of RIG is 20 I.U./kg (approximately 9 I.U./lb body weight). If possible, up to half the dose of RIG should be infiltrated in the area about the wound and the rest administered intramuscularly. When ARS must be used, the recommended dose is 40 I.U./kg (approximately 18 I.U./lb or 1 vial of 1000 I.U./55 lb body weight).

Local pain and low grade fever may follow RIG administration. ARS produces serum sickness in about 40 percent of adults with a lower reaction rate in children. Sensitivity to horse serum should be evaluated prior to administration of ARS in the manner described previously for equine antiserum in this chapter.

The two rabies vaccines used in the United States are human diploid cell rabies vaccine (HDCV) and the duck embryo vaccine (DEV). Lilly Laboratories ceased production of DEV in 1982. Both are inactivated virus vaccines and supplied in 1 ml single dose vials of lyophilized vaccine with accompanying diluent. HDCV should be used whenever available as only five doses are necessary for treatment as opposed to 14 to 21 doses of DEV.

Adverse reactions to HDCV consist of erythema, swelling, and itching at the injection site in about 25 percent of patients and systemic symptoms such as headache, abdominal pain, muscle aches, and dizziness occur in 20 percent of patients. Systemic allergic reactions have also been reported.

Local reactions to DEV are very common. Most patients experience pain, erythema, and induration at the injection site. Systemic symptoms occur in 33 percent after five to eight doses. Anaphylaxis occurs in less than 1 percent but can occur after the first dose in persons sensitized to avian tissue. Rare neuroparalytic reactions occur.

Bites by Venenating Arthropods

Spiders

Of all the spiders, the black widow or *Lactrodectus mactans* deserves special mention. It is present thoughout the United States and is frequently found in refuse heaps or near stables. The female is one-half inch long, coal black, and shiny, and has a red or orange hour-glass on her ventral surface. Her bite produces two tiny red punctures. The usual symptoms are pain at the time of the bite that becomes severe in about 30 minutes. This is followed by tremor, muscular rigidity of the abdomen, restlessness, and nausea. Headache, dizziness, and a rise in blood pressure may also occur. The outcome depends upon the physical status of the patient, the amount of toxin injected, and the rapidity with which treatment is started. The venom is neurotoxic, resulting in ascending paralysis and damage to the peripheral nerve endings.

Specific antivenin neutralizes the toxin in 30 to 60 minutes reducing the convalescent period and mortality rate. The antivenin (Lysovar®, Merck, Sharpe and Dohme) is also a horse serum product and sensitivity testing must be conducted as previously described. It is administered intramuscularly.

Cold compresses or ice packs on or about the local bite or application of Triamcenolone cream® 0.1 percent ointment will help control the pain. Dyspnea and muscular spasms should be treated with Diazepam, 5-10 mg, and with a slow intravenous infusion of 10 ml of a 10 percent solution of calcium gluconate which may be repeated at four hour intervals as necessary. Severe pain may respond to acetaminophen or meperidine.

The brown recluse spider (*Loxosceles Reclusa*) lives in cellars and barns. This spider has a violin-shaped mark on its back. The bite may be painless, but more often the reaction starts with edema and progreses in 24 hours through bulla formation, ischemia, cyanosis, and finally necrosis.

If the local reaction to a brown recluse spider bite or a bite due to an unidentified spider progresses over 8-12 hours to bulla formation or ischemia, the patient should be treated with high dose prednisone for one week (1 mg/kg/day). Corticosteroids (Triamcinolone acetonide suspension 5 mg/ml 1-2 ml total volume) injected into the lesion may be used when the bite is less than 12 hours old.

After initial evaluation and treatment, a patient having systemic reactions to an insect or spider bite should be transferred for treatment to the nearest local hospital. It is strongly advisable to obtain dermatologic and plastic surgery consultation because it is sometimes necessary to excise necrotic lesions that result from brown recluse spider bites, and this in turn is followed by skin grafts.

Tarantula bites cause no systemic reactions, but locally the reactions may be severe, especially in children. The wound should be cleansed thoroughly with soap and water and debrided if necessary. Local infiltration with an anesthetic (procaine and epinephrine) will relieve pain.

Tetanus toxoid or tetanus immune globulin and prophylactic antibiotics are indicated.

Ticks and Mites

The most notorious of the mites are the chiggers or "red bug" and the rat mite. The local lesion at the site of attachment can be treated by applying corticosteroids or lotions containing 1/4 percent menthol or 1/2 percent phenol.

The bite of several species of ticks may produce a flaccid ascending motor paralysis. This ascending paralysis begins in the lower extremities. Recovery is rapid and complete if the tick is removed. If not, the ascending paralysis may involve the muscles of respiration and death will result. The head of the tick should be removed surgically, if necessary. Supportive measures are also indicated. (See Shock, Chapter XII.)

Centipedes

The bite of a centipede causes a slight inflammatory reaction. Treatment is symptomatic.

Scorpions

The bite of most species produces only a local tissue reaction, while those found in the southwestern United States, *Centruroides sculpturatus*, produce a neurotoxic venom. The venom is elaborated in the swollen caudal segment (telson) which contains coupled poison glands and a stinger which it thrusts into its prey.

The symptoms produced by this scorpion bite produce local pain, extreme and perpetual restlessness, and roving eye movements. Children over ten years of age complain more of local pain and have less restlessness. Symptoms persist for three to thirty hours. Hypertension, respiratory distress, excess salivation, blurring vision, and slurred speech are also described.

Treatment consists of local application of ice to reduce pain. More extensive cryotherapy is not helpful. Triamcenolone ointment (0.1 percent) should be applied locally for the pruritis. An antivenin produced in goats is available in Arizona. Phenobarbital or diazepam have been used to control the agitation or restlessness, but sedatives should be used cautiously as excessive dosage has resulted in respiratory arrest.

Bites by Gila Monsters

Gila monster bites are rare and primarily caused by those in captivity. The symptoms of pain at the site occur within five minutes following the bite and may spread to involve the entire hand or foot within ten minutes with the duration variable. Edema progresses slowly with weakness or dizziness as common complaints. Local cleansing of the wound is indicated with removal of any teeth. There is no antivenin commercially available. Pain is controlled by aspirin, codeine, or meperidine. Appropriate antitetanus therapy is indicated, and antibiotic therapy is optional.

References

Russell, F. E. *Snake Venom Poisoning*. Philadelphia, J. B. Lippincott Co., 1980.

"Treatment of Snakebite in the U.S.A." The Medical Letter 24:87, Oct. 1, 1982.

Russell, F. E. "Snake Venom Poisoning in the United States." *Annual Revue of Medicine*: 31:247, 1980.

Arnold, R. E. *What to Do About Bites and Stings of Venomous Animals*. New York, Collier Books, 1974.

Rimsza, M. E., Zimmerman, D. R., and Bergeson, P. S. "Scorpion Envenomation." *Pediatrics* 66:298, 1980.

Rabies Prevention. Morbidity and Mortality Weekly Report. 29:265, June 13, 1980.

Chapter XII

THE ROLE OF THE CAMP HEALTH SUPERVISOR IN EMERGENCIES

Fortunately, life-threatening emergencies are rarely seen in summer camps. Nevertheless, the Health Supervisor may be confronted by a camper in severe shock, coma, convulsions, and cardiac or respiratory arrest. What should the treatment be for a camper with a severe burn, serious chest injury, or head or leg fracture? The Health Supervisor should be well-versed in emergency first aid measures so that his/her course of action will be correct and accomplished with dispatch before the camper is transported to a hospital for further treatment. The counselors should be well acquainted with the use of first aid measures in emergencies. A good camp director makes certain of this in the precamp orientation of his/her staff. This section will be devoted to a discussion of some of these emergencies so that the Health Supervisor will have a ready, on-the-spot reference and be prepared to direct rapid emergency measures should disaster strike.

Syncope Due to Heat

This is precipitated in unacclimatized persons after severe exercise or prolonged standing in excessive heat. When the outside temperature exceeds body temperature, a considerable portion of the circulating blood is diverted to the vessels of the skin to help maintain normal body temperature. If the patient's blood volume is not adequate for this adjustment, the venous return is poor, the pulse rises, blood pressure falls, and the patient faints. Response to rest in a horizontal position is immediate, and syncope is not likely to recur after acclimatization.

Heat Exhaustion (Sunstroke)

Heat exhaustion and heat cramps are manifestations of disorders of water and electrolyte metabolism and may occur in acclimatized individuals who overwork in a heated environment. The muscular cramps are reflections of salt depletion of the extracellular fluid because of inadequate intake of fluid and subsequent dehydration. The patient is able to perspire and maintain an approximately normal temperature. The patient's skin will be pale, clammy, and cool, and there will be generalized weakness. Nausea and vomiting are common. The blood pressure will be low and the pulse weak and fast. The pupils will be dilated, and the patient may be stuporous and may lapse into coma.

The patient should be treated by loosening the clothing and offering fluids *ad lib* if the patient is able to swallow. Parenteral fluids should be administered if the patient cannot take oral liquids.

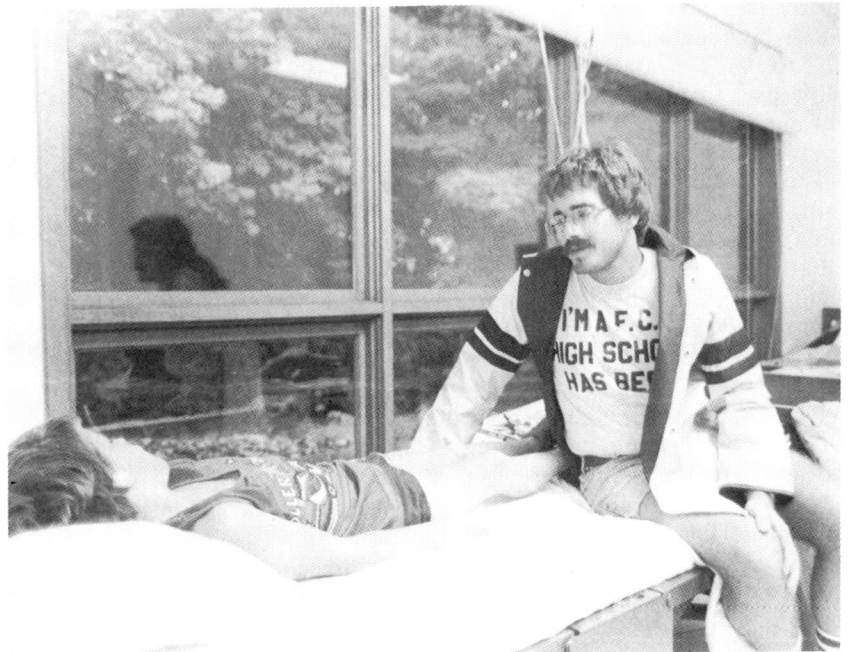

Heat Cramps

The patient is pale and perspires profusely. He complains of nausea and dizziness, extreme thirst, and severe abdominal cramps. The pulse is rapid but strong, and the body temperature may be slightly elevated. There may be muscle twitching or, in some instances, generalized convulsions. The patient should be allowed to rest in a cool place. Usually the patient will recover without being hospitalized. Fluids should be given orally. If there is marked dehydration, a normal saline solution should be given intravenously.

Heat Stroke (Heat Retention)

There is experimental evidence that with prolonged work or exercise in the heat there is a progressive decrease in the ability to perspire once the body temperature begins to rise. At a critical point, the body sweating mechanism may fail entirely.

The attack may have a sudden onset or the patient may give a history of diminution or absence of sweating during the preceding hours.

The patient will complain of a sensation of extreme heat and headache. The gait may be unsteady, and there may be mental confusion. The patient may be in a coma. The skin is hot and dry. The dryness of the skin is pathognomonic of heat stroke. The temperature at first may be 102° to 103°F, and then may climb quickly to 110°F. The breathing will be deep at first, then shallow, and finally Cheyne-Stokes in character. The pupils are dilated, and there may be generalized twitching, maniacal behavior, or generalized convulsions.

The patient may die immediately or within the first 24 hours. The unfavorable presenting manifestations are a temperature over 106°F, coma, hypotension, uremia, and hyperkalemia.

Pathologic findings at autopsy are cerebral edema and petechial hemorrhages in the hypothalamus.

Obviously, heroic measures are indicated if the patient is to survive. Strip the patient, wrap him in wet towels and ventilate with an electric fan. Measures should be instituted to combat shock and control convulsions (see entries in this chapter). If the body temperature falls to 101° to 102°F, cooling should be stopped. It is important to rub the extremities and body vigorously in an effort to stimulate circulation to the skin. If the body temperature falls and perspiration appears, the outcome may be favorable. The patient may then be transferred to a hospital for further therapy. There is no evidence that permanent residuals result from heat stroke, such as persistent intolerance to heat or neurologic signs of permanent brain damage.

Anaphylaxis

An anaphylactic reaction is a precipitous, unexpected disaster where the physician has to be ready for instantaneous action if the victim is to be saved. Anaphylaxis is a relatively rare emergency, but there are indications that it is seen with increasingly greater frequency. Despite appropriate therapy, it has been reported that 10 percent of anaphylactic reactions end fatally.

Many substances have been incriminated, including the antibiotics and antiserums such as equine tetanus antitoxin.

The clinical picture of anaphylaxis may be sudden collapse and cardiorespiratory arrest. The usual sequence is the development of apprehension by the patient, nausea, diaphoresis, and a pounding headache. Dyspnea develops with or without wheezing, cyanosis, circulatory collapse, and coma. Convulsions may also occur. Before circulatory collapse, the patient may develop severe pruritis and urticaria, followed by angioneurotic edema.

The best approach to therapy would be prevention, but this is easier said than done. Certain precautions should be kept in mind.

Always obtain a complete history about any allergic tendency.

Since oral administration of drugs may produce less frequent and less severe reactions, this should be the preferred method of administering drugs in a camp. It should be pointed out, however, that fatal anaphylactic reactions have been reported even after oral administration of drugs.

Patients who are receiving allergen extracts for atopic hyposensitization should be kept in the infirmary for 15 to 20 minutes after the injection so that if a reaction occurs the physician and nurse will be there to administer emergency therapy.

Preliminary "skin testing" with the potential anaphylactogen should be done, although a negative test does not insure against an anaphylactic reaction, and anaphylactic reactions have been reported after such tests. A positive reaction should alert the physician so that he proceeds with caution (see Chapter XI).

The Health Supervisor must be prepared to act quickly; 0.3-0.5 ml of 1:1000 epinephrine should be given intramuscularly immediately. A tourniquet should be placed above the site of the injection of the offending substance if this has been given into an extremity, and an additional 0.25 ml of epinephrine should be given into the site.

If there is no immediate improvement, aqueous (epinephrine 1:100 diluted in physiologic saline 1:10 and 0.01 mg/kg) should be given intravenously. The total dose of epinephrine should not exceed 0.5 ml and should be given slowly. The epinephrin may be repeated in 5-15 minutes. An infusion of physiologic saline should be started and metaraminal bitartrate (Aramine®) might be given and positive pressure oxygen administered. If circulatory collapse develops, the treatment should be instituted as described under "Shock" in this chapter. If urticaria develops or edema appears, particularly edema of the larynx, an intramuscular injection of diphenhydramine hydrochloride (Bendadryl®) can be given (25-50 mg over a 10-15 minute period). Some experts advise the use of 100-200 mg of hydrocortisone intravenously immediately and repeated every 4-6 hours as required.

Burns

The depth of the burn is important from a prognostic standpoint. One classifies burns as follows:

1. Superficial (first degree)—there is only erythema.
2. Partial skin thickness (second degree)—there is bleb formation.
3. Deep (third degree)—the full thickness of the skin is involved and/or the subcutaneous or deeper tissues. There may be discoloration and charring.

Shock is much more common if the head, face, hands, genitalia, and feet are burned. The severity of the pain will be much greater if the face, hands, or flexion creases and joint areas are involved.

The longer the interval between the burn and treatment the greater the danger from shock and infection. Children under five years and elderly individuals have a poor prognosis in severe burns.

The emergency treatment involves a quick decision as to whether the patient will need hospitalization or not. This can be determined immediately.

If a burn is superficial (first degree) and localized, and involves less than 20 percent of the body surface, the following steps should be taken:

1. Wash thoroughly with nonmedicated soap and water.
2. Apply Betadyne® ointment dressing.
3. Aspirin should be given for pain, or a barbiturate should be administered as a sedative.
4. Tetanus toxoid should be given if the burn is dirty.

If the burn is severe and greater than 20 percent, pain and restlessness should be controlled by subcutaneous or intramuscular administration of a barbiturate and/or morphine or Demerol® , and the patient should be prepared for transfer to the appropriate hospital facility.

Shock

Shock may be caused by a severe burn, massive hemmorhage, severe crushing injury, traumatic amputation, major fracture, a chest wound which penetrates the pleura, and abdominal wounds.

This type of surgical or traumatic shock is brought on by a sudden reduction in the volume of circulating blood. The venous pressure is reduced and thus the diastolic filling of the heart is also reduced. The cardiac output falls, but the blood pressure is maintained for a time by a reflex arteriolar constriction. The blood flow progressively diminishes, and the arteriolar constriction fails to maintain the blood pressure, and generalized tissue hypoxia ensues.

The symptoms and signs of shock are very striking. The patient is prostrated but usually conscious, the skin is moist, and there may be slight cyanosis; the pulse is rapid and feeble, and the extremities are cold and clammy. The patient is often obtunded and may be restless and complain of thirst; there is progressive hypotension, and as the hypoxia of the tissues increases, metabolic acidosis develops.

The longer this precarious state exists, the worse the prognosis. It is vital, therefore, that the treatment of shock take precedence after the control of gross hemorrhage and the provision of adequate oxygenation.

The patient should be kept comfortable and warm. In very severe shock, the foot of the bed should be elevated. In head injuries, or if there is pulmonary distress, the head should be raised slightly. Oxygen should be administered by face mask under positive pressure, and there should be available solutions of normal saline or 5 percent glucose in saline which should be started intravenously and continued enroute to the hospital. If the veins are collapsed, a cut down should be done. The patient should have a blood pressure cuff upon his arm so that the pressure can be monitored every two or three minutes while any of the following vasoconstrictive agents are given.

Metaramine bitartrate (Aramine®) may be given intravenously, intramuscularly, or subcutaneously. This rarely causes sloughing of tissues if extravasation occurs. If it is difficult to get into a vein, the drug may be given intramuscularly (2-10 mg). If an infusion of glucose in saline has been started, the drug may be given (15-100 mg in 1000 ml of solution). The rate and the amount administered is determined by the blood pressure response. The intramuscular route will give a response in seven to ten minutes; the intravenous administration in one to two minutes. The preferred course of action in camp would be to start the infusion of saline or glucose in saline and administer the Aramine® intramuscularly.

The physician may prefer other vasoconstrictive agents such as phenylephrine hydrochloride (Neo-Synephrine®). The dose is 3-5 mg added to 500-1000 ml of solution which is dripped in slowly while the blood pressure is monitored every two minutes. Ephedrine sulfate may be used in a dose of 10-25 mg in 500-1000 ml of solution which is dripped in slowly. Here, also, the blood pressure should be monitored. Arterenol bitartrate (Levophed®, norepinephrine) may be preferred and this may be given in a dose of 4 mg in 1000 ml of solution. The blood pressure should be monitored every two minutes. It should be remembered that extensive necrosis may occur if the drug extravasates into the tissues.

Pain should be controlled by the administration of morphine sulfate. This should not be used in severe chest or head injuries because of its respiratory depressant effects. In cases of severe shock which do not respond to the above measures, hydrocortisone sodium succinate (Solu-Cortef®) 100 mg may be given intravenously and repeated in four hours. The hospital should be called and alerted about the patient's arrival, and the Health Supervisor should accompany the patient to the hospital. The oxygen and fluid infusion could be administered enroute.

In case of a severe burn, the clothing should be removed gently from the burned areas and the burned areas should be washed gently with soap and water. No extensive debridement should be attempted, nor should blebs be opened.

If the burn is extensive, and until hospitalization can be provided, pads of sterile gauze should be applied and then the patient covered with a sheet. Splints should be applied to prevent motion of the burned areas.

Tetanus toxoid or tetanus immune globulin (human) may be given after the patient is in the hospital, and the patient should be started upon prophylactic antibiotics.

Electrical Burns

When electric current passes through living tissue, damage may be more severe than is apparent. Immediate death may occur from ventricular fibrillation. Respiratory arrest may occur. Low tension currents are more dangerous than high tension, and alternating current is more dangerous than direct current. The points of entrance and exit should be identified, and in this way some idea of the kind of tissue damage can be gained. The patient should be moved away from the wire or appliance with a dry wooden pole. The operator should wear insulated gloves. If the patient is not breathing, artificial respiration should be started and the patient handled in very much the same way as outlined under the section on cardiac arrest which appears later in this chapter.

Chest Injuries

Acute restlessness and anxiety may be the only manifestations of alveolar and/or mediastinal bleeding in a patient with a history of severe compresssion injury of the thorax. The patient will be in shock, and the treatment as outlined under "Shock" should be followed. The chest should not be taped, because this will limit aeration, and narcotics should not be used because of the danger of respiratory depression.

If a tension pneumothorax is suspected and verified by physical examination, a No. 10 or No. 18 needle should be inserted between the second and third ribs in the midclavicular line. The upper margin of the lower rib in the intercostal space should be used as a guide to avoid nicking the intercostal artery. A finger cot should be fastened to the base of the needle, and a small hole should be made in the tip of the cot. This device will serve as a flutter valve as the patient is transported to the hospital.

If the pleura is lacerated by a knife or bullet wound or if there is a compound rib fracture, cover the surface laceration with petroleum jelly and a pressure bandage. The patient should be given oxygen, either by mask or intranasal catheter, and treated for shock while being transferred to a hospital.

Fractures

In all cases of severe trauma where a fracture is suspected, a roentgenogram should be obtained. If the injury is severe enough, shock may be present and treatment as outlined under "Shock" should be instituted.

Campers who sustain fractures of any kind should be transferred for definitive treatment to a hospital. It is advisable to get an orthopedic opinion even if the fracture involves a finger or toe.

Head Injuries

When there is the possibility of a fracture, brain concussion, or intracranial hemorrhage, the camper should be given emergency first-aid therapy and transferred to a hospital for further diagnostic work and treatment.

By quick examination, the Health Supervisor should determine the extent of the injury and institute the necessary emergency first-aid measures.

The Health Supervisor should do a careful neurologic examination and pay particular attention to evidence of bleeding from the ears, nose, and throat (basilar skull fracture). The mental status of the patient should be determined. Is the patient oriented? Does he have any memory of the accident? The reflexes can be checked quickly, and sensory and motor loss should be determined. This examination will serve as a standard of reference for subsequent examinations at the hospital.

The blood pressure, pulse, respiration, and adequacy of the airway should be checked. An adequate airway may be achieved by supporting the angles of the jaw. If the patient is vomiting, he should be turned on his side to prevent aspiration. If the patient is in shock, emergency treatment should be initiated at once as described under "Shock."

Opiates should be avoided in head injuries because of their effect on the pupillary reaction and depression of the respiratory center. If there are associated severe injuries and the pain is intense, codeine may be given cautiously. It should be administered parenterally in half the recommended dose. Sedation should also be avoided unless there is extreme restlessness or if the patient is in an excited state. The drugs of choice are sodium phenobarbital or chloral hydrate.

The patient should be moved with caution, keeping it in mind that there may be cervical, dorsal, or lumbar spine injury. Sandbags or rolled blankets should be placed upon either side of the patient for immobilization.

If the patient is cyanotic or dyspneic, oxygen should be administered by mask. The patient should not be given anything by mouth. It is advisable for the Health Supervisor to accompany the patient to the hospital and monitor the pulse, respiration, blood pressure, and state of consciousness enroute.

The Health Supervisor should watch for deepening coma and depression of the gag and corneal reflexes. Onset of paralysis and progressive development of stupor with a dilated pupil which is nonreactive to light are grave signs, as are a drop in pulse rate and the onset of irregular respiration. The above manifestations make the prognosis very serious and increase the probability of surgical intervention.

Neck and Spinal Cord Injuries

Severe neck injury should always be suspected whenever there is direct trauma to the head or neck, especially if the neck was bent at the time of injury. Any story involving automobile collision, especially if there is a sudden jerk ("whiplash injury"), deserves careful examination, especially if the patient complains of severe pain or sensory disturbance in the back of the head, or the neck, shoulders, or arms.

Where the index of suspicion is high that one is dealing with either a fracture or dislocation, the patient should be transferred to a hospital. The head should be immobilized by sandbags or pillows on either side so that there is as little neck movement as possible, and the Health Supervisor should accompany the patient. The driver should avoid speed or rough roads to keep the jarring down to a minimum.

"Whiplash injury" sustained during automobile accidents may not produce symptoms for one to three days, and there may be extensive soft tissue hemorrhage. Sometimes the soft tissue injury may cause acute symptoms out of proportion to the trauma sustained. It is sometimes difficult to differentiate this kind of injury from a fracture or dislocation. X-rays of the cervical spine and an opinion from a neurosurgeon should be obtained in all instances of moderately severe neck injuries.

All severe injuries to the head, neck, or back should be considered as possible spinal cord injuries. When the Health Supervisor arrives on the scene, he/she should examine the patient and keep the following points in mind. Acute flexion or hypertension injuries are more likely to cause cord damage. Radicular pain is common with cord injuries so that the localization of the pain is important. The spine should be palpated carefully from the base of the skull down and any deformity or prominence of a spinous process looked for. Muscle spasm, pain, or tenderness may also help the Health Supervisor to localize the injury. Motion of the extremities should be checked as well as reflexes and sensory response to light, touch, and pin prick. The patient may need morphine for pain; or the patient may be in shock, and immediate therapy should be instituted for this. The patient should, of course, be transferred to a hospital for diagnostic studies and therapy. The Health Supervisor should personally supervise the lifting of the patient onto the spine board, and the spine should be immobilized with sandbags, pillows, or blankets. Careful, gentle handling must be stressed. The driver of the vehicle should proceed slowly, avoiding rough roads.

Drowning

Mucous should be removed from the mouth and throat by turning the head to the side and sweeping it out with the finger. Constricting clothing should be removed as quickly as possible.

There should be immediate institution of resuscitation. Aquatic personnel should be well-versed in these methods and will have started emergency treatment before the camp Health Supervisor arrives on the scene. If mechanical resuscitation equipment is available, this should be used. If breathing has been reestablished, the patient should be transferred to a hospital. Antibiotics should be given prophylactically. Respiratory and cardiac stimulants are of little value until spontaneous respiration has been reestablished.

Choking on Food

In the event that a camper chokes on food and cannot speak, cough, or breathe, give four quick back blows followed by four upward and inward abdominal or chest thrusts. For the abdominal thrust, grasp one fist with

Figure 9
Chest Thrust, Standing

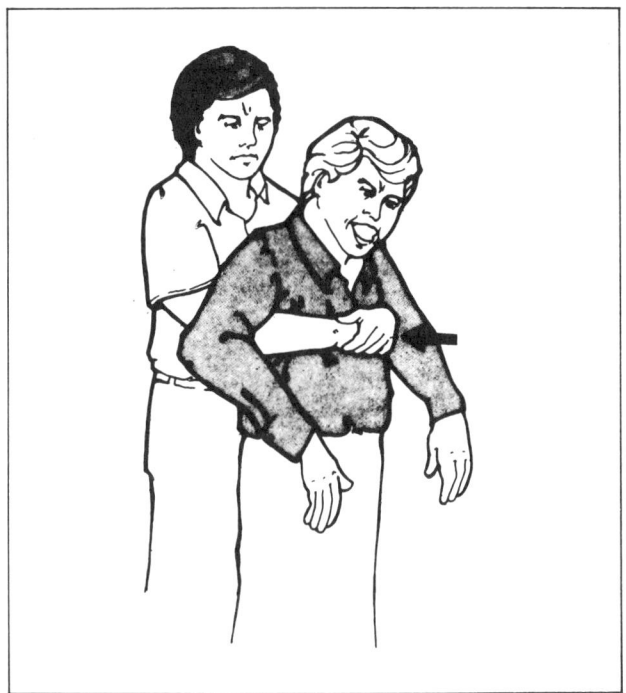

your other hand with the thumb side of your fist in the midline of the rib cage, and slightly above the waist. For the chest thrust, use the same hand position, but place the arms further up the midline of the rib cage as shown in *Figure 9*.

Emergency Tracheotomy

This procedure would indeed be a rarity in a camp situation. Such an emergency procedure would be necessary if a foreign body becomes lodged in the larynx or trachea. Inflammatory or allergic reactions would be unlikely causes for an on-the-spot tracheotomy. If there is impending danger of asphyxiation, then an emergency tracheotomy should be performed. The head of the patient should be hyperextended with a towel under the cervical spine. The trachea is fixed between the thumb and forefinger of one hand, and a vertical incision is made approximately midway between the cricoid cartilage and suprasternal notch. The strip muscles and facia are cut until the trachea is reached. Two or three tracheal rings are cut well below the cricoid cartilage. The trachea may be kept open by any kind of tube such as stethoscope tubing. The wound should be packed for hemostasis, and the Health Supervisor should accompany the patient to the nearest hospital for further treatment.

Convulsion

The occurrence of an isolated, initial, convulsive episode would be extremely rare at camp. It is possible that heat stroke may precipitate this. Febrile convulsions may be ushered in by overwhelming bacterial sepsis and meningitis. The convulsions may be the first manifestations of a space-occupying lesion in the brain. The emergency treatment is quite simple, and the camper should be transferred to the hospital or home for further diagnostic procedures and therapy. The emergency measures which should be taken are as follows.

The camper should be protected from injury by gentle restraint and the clothing about the neck should be loosened. The patient should be turned on his side so that he does not aspirate pooled secretions or vomitus. If suction is available, this should be used to aspirate secretions, and if oxygen is available, this should be administered. Sponging with tepid water should be started if the patient has fever. Sodium phenobarbital may be administered (see Appendix II for dosage), and the intramuscular route should be the one of choice at camp. The intravenous route may be hazardous if the administration of the drug is not slow and cautious, because respiratory arrest may ensue and complicate the situation. Another barbiturate which may be used is Seconal® (see Appendix II for dosage). If an overwhelming infection is suspected, the patient should receive parenteral pencillin before transfer to a hospital. (See page 59, Seizure Disorder.)

Cardiac Arrest

If the patient is in coma or is not breathing, emergency resuscitation measures take precedence over everything else. It is imperative that the following should be tried. (The following description of cardiopulmonary resuscitation (CPR) was taken from the manual prepared by the American Heart Association. Also refer to *Figure 10* and *Tables VIII* and *IX* which were prepared by the American Heart Association and portrays this emergency procedure.)

Place the patient in the supine position. Determine quickly if there is any airway obstruction by finger palpitation. If there is fluid or vomitus in the pharynx or nose, the head of the patient should be turned to the side and the chest elevated to allow the fluid to run out. The head should then be placed in overextension by a pad or towel under the lower cervical spine. The operator should be to one side of the patient.

The heel of one hand should be placed over the lower sternum and the other hand on top of it. Firm pressure is applied vertically downward with the operator's body weight as the compressing force. The down-

Figure 10
Cardiopulmonary Resuscitation (CPR)

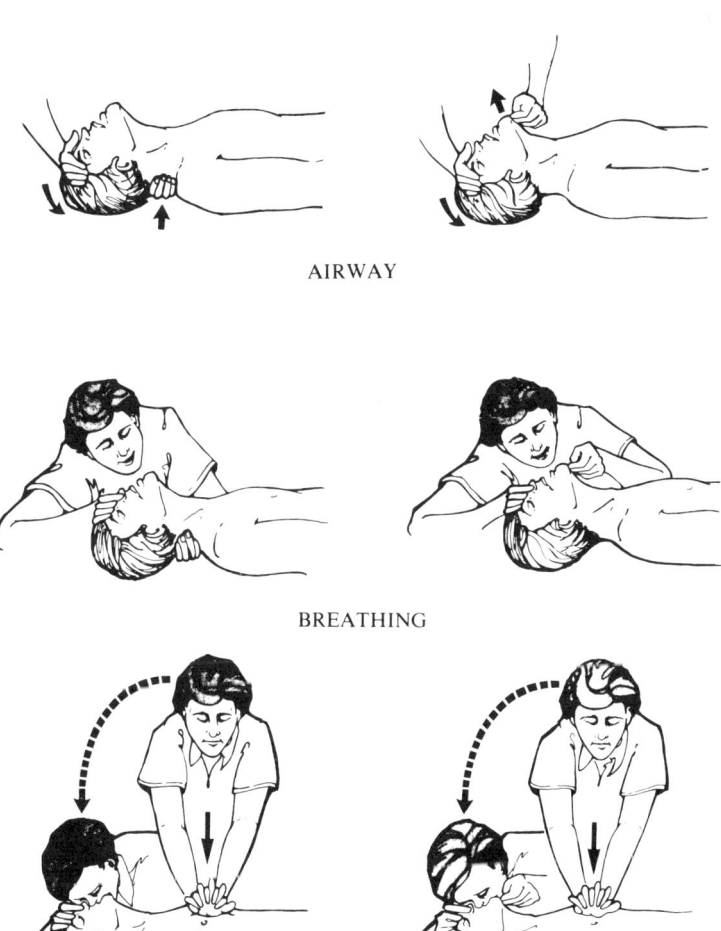

ward pressure should be applied about 60 to 70 times per minute. The sternum should move downward one to two inches when pressure is applied. The pressure should be relaxed after each compression to allow the heart to fill with blood.

A second person could be quickly instructed to start mouth-to-mouth resuscitation. One hand is placed under the neck and the head is over-extended. The chin should then be pulled forward. He/she then places

Table VIII
American Heart Association
Cardiopulmonary Resuscitation and Emergency Cardiac Care
Rationale for Two Rescuer CPR

ELAPSED TIME (Seconds) Min.	Max.	ACTIVITY AND TIME (Seconds)	CRITICAL PERFORMANCE	RATIONALE
		1st rescuer resumes CPR. 2nd rescuer identifies himself and checks pulse for effective compressions.	Technique for single rescuer. 2nd rescuer says, "I know how to do CPR." Fingers palpate for carotid pulse.	To locate the carotid pulse.
		2nd rescuer calls out, "Stop compressions" and checks for spontaneous pulse and breathing. (5 sec.)	Five second pause to check for spontaneous pulse and breathing. 2nd rescuer should inform the 1st rescuer of the status of the victim and the need for either ventilations, compressions or both. Says, "No pulse, continue CPR."	Provides a second assessment of pulse and breathing and the need for CPR.
		2nd rescuer ventilates once.	Ventilates properly and observes chest rise.	
		1st rescuer resumes compressions.	Two-rescuer rate and ratio.	2nd rescuer ventilation triggers change of rate and ratio.
		Minimum of two cycles of 5 compressions and 1 ventilation. (8-10 sec.) Switch and repeat until examiner is satisfied.	Correct rate of compressions.	
			Says mnemonic.	Necessary to establish rhythm.
			Interposes breath.	
			No pause for ventilation.	
			Calls for switch.	Signal for change must be clear.
			Switches.	
			Switches back.	
			Checks pulse (by ventilator).	
			Technique as above.	

(Left bracket label: TWO RESCUERS)

Table IX
American Heart Association
Cardiopulmonary Resuscitation and Emergency Cardiac Care
Rationale for One Rescuer CPR

ELAPSED TIME (seconds) Min.	Max.	ACTIVITY AND TIME (seconds)	CRITICAL PERFORMANCE	RATIONALE
4	10	Establish unresponsiveness and call out for help. Allow 4-10 sec. if face down and turning is required.	Tap, gently shake shoulder and shout, "Are you OK?" Call out, "Help!" Turn if necessary.	Frequently victim will be face down. Effective external chest compression can only be provided with victim flat on back on a hard surface.
			Adequate time.	Accurate diagnosis is important. Four to ten seconds gives time to do that and to review mentally the sequence of CPR.
7	15	Open airway. Establish breathlessness. (Look, Listen, and Feel) (3-5 sec.)	Kneels properly	
			Head tilt with one hand on forehead and neck lift or chin lift with other hand.	Airway must be opened to establish breathlessness. Many victims may be making respiratory efforts that are ineffective because of obstruction.
			Ear over mouth, observe chest	
10	20	Four ventilations. (3-5 sec.)	Ventilate properly 4 times and observe chest rise.	
15	30	Establish pulse and stimulate activation of EMS system. (5-10 sec.)	Fingers palpate for carotid pulse on near side (other hand on forehead maintains head tilt).	This activity should take 5-10 seconds, because not only does it take time to find the right place, but the pulse may be very slow or very weak and rapid.

Table IX (continued)

			Know local EMS number.	EMS is activated at this time so information on breathing and pulse can be given to dispatcher.
			Adequate time.	
69	96	Four cycles of 15 compressions and 2 ventilations. (54-68 sec.)	Proper body position	
			Landmark check each time.	
			Position of hands.	Precision in hand placement is essential to avoid serious injury.
			Vertical compression.	
			Says mnemonic.	Necessary to establish rhythm.
			Proper rate.	Should attempt to accomplish 60 compressions and 9 ventilations per minute.
			Proper ratio.	
			No bouncing.	
			Ventilates properly.	
72	101	Check for return of and spontaneous breathing. (3-5 sec.)	Check pulse and breathing.	

his/her mouth over the patient's mouth, forcibly inflates the lungs, and then removes his/her mouth to allow the patient to exhale passively. These inhalations should follow each relaxation of the sternal compression.

A third person should be dispatched for emergency vehicle transportation, or the patient could be quickly transferred to a station wagon and the resuscitative measures continued on the way to the hospital.

The physician does not know whether the heart of the patient is asystolic or in a state of fibrillation. If spontaneous contraction of the heart appears within one or two minutes and there is a palpable pulse, the heart was probably in asystole. If this does not occur, the heart is either atonic or fibrillating. An electrocardiogram will distinguish between these two states, but this is not available at camp. Also, if the heart is fibrillating, an external defibrillator should be used. The electrodes should be applied firmly, one over the cardiac apex, the other over the sternal notch. Apply the shock; do not touch the patient or allow anyone else to touch the patient when applying the shock. Try a shock of 440 volts AC at 0.25 seconds. If this is ineffective, try three shocks in rapid succession.

If the fibrillation persists, epinephrine should be injected into the left ventricle (0.2 ml of 1:1000 solution of epinephrine mixed with 10 ml of normal saline). Five ml of a 10 percent solution of $CaCl_2$ might be given intravenously. Cardiac compression should be maintained after the shocks and certainly after defibrillation. An electrocardiograph and defibrillator will not be available in camp; these instruments and emergency medications should be made available immediately upon arrival at the hospital.

How long should cardiac compression and oral resuscitation be continued? This is difficult to answer, but if there is no response in an hour, the chances of survival are remote.*

I would not recommend open cardiac massage in a camp situation. The key points to remember are not to delay the institution of the above resuscitative measures. Both cardiac compression and oral resuscitation are important. The lungs must be aerated and effective circulation must be maintained. *The patient should be transported to a hospital as soon as possible, and these emergency measures can be continued en route.*

Artificial respiration should be continued for at least four hours before declaring the patient dead. The Health Supervisor should remem-

---

*The usual criteria for death are:

1. The absence of pulse beat and the absence of heart beat and breath sounds as determined by stethoscopic examination;
2. The absence of fogging of a mirror held over the face;
3. The absence of corneal reflex;
4. Rigor mortis and dependent cyaosis;
5. Flat base line of the electrocardiographic tracing.

ber that the usual criteria for death do not apply following electric shock. Breathing has been reestablished eight hours after an electric shock.

In camp, it is not necessary to keep prolonged artificial respiration. Provisions can be made for the camper to be transferred to a hospital and artificial respiration can be continued while en route.

It would be advisable for the camp director to require that all counselors take the course in cardiopulmonary resuscitation (CPR) before coming to camp. These courses are given at local Heart Associations, YMCA's, and fire stations so that it is quite easy to earn a certificate in CPR.

Malpractice

It is quite certain that the Health Supervisor might be concerned about legal action because of alleged improper emergency treatment received by a camper.

Malpractice suits are usually based on accusations of negligence upon the part of the Health Supervisor which result in injury to the patient. Negligence may consist of the omission of proper and recognized methods of examination and treatment or the use of improper and generally unacceptable methods of examination and treatment.

Recognized methods of treatment and examination vary in different localities. A Health Supervisor is required to use knowledge, skill, and methods common to other medical personnel practicing under similar circumstances. A general practitioner is not expected to possess the skill and knowledge of a specialist in a medical center. It should also be pointed out that the statute of limitations is defined as the time that the patient or their parents in the case of a minor become aware of the injury and not from the date of the supposed negligent act which resulted in the injury.

The impression that a lesser standard of care is acceptable in emergencies is not true. The legal definition of a physician's obligations in emergency situations might well be summed up in this statement:

> A physician is required to excercise or use such reasonable and ordinary care, skill, and diligence as a physician in good standing in the same area in the same general line of practice ordinarily uses in like cases.

The following precautions should be taken by the Health Supervisor to protect himself/herself: First, all Health Supervisors should be adequately covered by malpractice insurance. The Health Supervisor must keep adequate written records (Chapter II, *Figure 8*) and should obtain competent consultation in problem cases. He should avoid the use of experimental or generally unacceptable procedures of treatment. The parents

Figure 11

Procedures for Serious Cases Involving Serious Illness or Injury

In case of serious injury or illness, parents should be notified immediately. This should be done by telephone whenever possible. Be careful not to frighten or excite them, but be factual and reassure them that everything possible is being done.

In Case of Serious Accident

Notify:
   Camp director
   Authorities—Police, Sheriff, etc.
   Parents
   Collect all facts, including names
     of witnesses

In Case of Serious Illness

Get the doctor
Alert a hospital
Arrange transportation
Notify health authorities if contagion is suspected;
   follow their instructions
Notify camp director

Special Note: Any time a camper or staff member is taken to a hospital or physician out of camp, the camper's Physical Examination and Health Record Form (or copies) should be delivered to the examining physician. (Be sure to retrieve them and return to the camp file.)

In Case of a Fatality

Notify local authorities. The police and coroner must institute an inquiry to determine the cause of death—whether reasonable precautions were taken to prevent the accident. This also will include a decision as to whether or not the usual practices of the camp were followed at the time of the accident.

Notify camp director as he/she must arrange to notify parents.

Get all facts, including statements of all witnesses.

Include information:

Who? Name of deceased, age.
When? Date, time of day.
Where? Location.
What? Nature of accident or illness.
How? (If known; i.e., swimming, hiking, boating, etc.)

Also inform American Camping Association, Bradford Woods, Martinsville, IN 46151.

should be completely informed about an accident and the extent of an injury. The consultant should also inform the parents. The American Camping Association has published a short list of valuable suggestions for operating procedures to follow by the physician, nurse, camp director, or counselor in cases involving serious illness or injury and this is reproduced with their permission in *Figure 11*.

References

Jackson, C. "Tracheostomy." Trans. Amer. Laryng. Rhinol. Otol. Soc., p. 337, 1909.

Appendix I

The Health Supervisor is in a critical position when confronted with the possibility of a communicable disease. Questions of communicability, quarantine, isolation, prophylaxis, and treatment are of paramount importance in the prevention of a possible epidemic in their camp.

Sore throat may be due to a Group A beta hemolytic streptococcus, infectious mononucleosis due to EB virus, or some other viral agent. At this time diphtheria is usually a remote possibility, though it still should be considered in the differential diagnosis.

Diseases which rarely would be seen are also included in this section, because they may be considered in the differential diagnoses in a number of febrile illnesses. Also, the common childhood diseases are included though most children and adolescents have received appropriate immunizations prior to entering elementary school and may have received boosters prior to coming to camp.

The Report of the Committee on Infectious Disease of the American Academy of Pediatrics has an excellent outline of many communicable diseases and was one of the sources of information for this section.

An attempt was made to abstract the most important and pertinent information about these diseases and to organize the discussion in brief outline form. It is hoped that this information will give the Health Supervisor sufficient information to recognize the disease, initiate therapy, and institute necessary precautions.

Disease	Incubation Period	Isolation	Prevention and Treatment
Amebiasis The primary site of the infection is the colon associated with abdominal discomfort. There is diarrhea alternating with constipation. Blood and mucus are present in the stool but little pus. Differential diagnosis includes shigellosis, appendicitis and ulcerative colitis. The causative agent is the *Entamoeba histolytica*. Diagnosis is made by identification of trophozoites or cysts of *Entamoeba histolytica* in the feces. The reservoir of infection is cysts from feces of infected persons. The infection is transmitted by eating contaminated vegetables (raw), or drinking contaminated water. The food may be contaminated by flies or by soiled hands of infected food handlers.	2 wks. or less when parasites appear in stool. Symptomatic onset unpredictable.	None. Infected person should be restricted from food handling.	Metronidazole: 35-50 mg/kg daily in 2-3 divided doses (max: 800 mg. t.i.d.) for 7 days for symptomatic dysentery. Tetracycline 30 mg/kg/day (max: 2 gm daily) for 7 days for asymptomatic (carrier) patients. Preventive measures: 1. Sanitary disposal of feces. 2. Protection of water supply. 3. Careful selection of food handlers. 4. Disinfect food by cooking and water by boiling or chlorination.
Arthropod-Borne Viral Infections **1) Encephalitis** The etiologic agents include Eastern equine, Western equine, Venezuelan equine, Powassen, St. Louis, and California encephalitis viruses. Each agent has variable geographic distribution in the United States and is transmitted through an arthropod vector (mosquito or tick). Life cycle is especially maintained through birds, horses, and rodents. This comprises a group of diseases which may involve the spinal cord, meninges, and brain resulting in meningeal, encephalitic, or meningoencephalitic symptoms. Headache, vomiting, fever, lethargy, stupor, disorientation, coma, tremors, spasticity, and convulsions may occur. There is a pleocytosis of 50-400 cells/ml, predominantly mononuclear. There is no direct communicability from man-to-man. A rise in specific antibody titer using hemagglutination-inhibiting, comple-	California: 5-15 days. Eastern equine: 5-15 days. Powassan: 4-18 days. St. Louis: 4-21 days. Venezuelan equine: 2-5 days. Western equine: 5-10 days.	None except Venezuelan equine—virus may be present 2-4 days in the nasopharynx.	There is no specific treatment. There is no specific vaccine available for those viral agents commonly causing the disease in North America.

ment fixation, fluorescent, or neutralization techniques are the usual means of demonstrating infection with these viruses.

2) Colorado Tick Fever
The etiologic agent is an orbivirus. This is an acute febrile illness which lasts for 2-3 days and may have an associated rash. There is a remission of 2-7 days and then a recurrence of fever for 2-10 days. The reservoir of infection is the tick, *Dermacentor andersoni*. The reservoir is in the blood of infected persons and in ticks because of transovarian passage. The ticks acquire infection through feeding on infected animals during a period of viremia and then pass this on to man during feeding. The disease is not transmitted from man-to-man and is seen in the Pacific Northwest and Rocky Mountain areas.

3-6 days.

None.

There is no specific treatment. Prevention is best accomplished by control of ticks.

Ascariasis
This is a common, chronic infection caused by the round worm, *Ascaris lumbricoides*. Heavy infection may produce digestive disturbances, abdominal pain, and sleeplessness. Live worms passed in the stool, or if found in the vomitus, are the first signs of infection. After ingestion, the embryonated eggs hatch in the intestine. Larvae penetrate the wall and reach the lungs by way of the lymphatic and circulatory systems. Most larvae, after reaching the lungs, pass into the air passages, then ascend the bronchi, are swallowed, and eventually reach the small intestine where they grow to maturity. The source of infection is the egg of Ascaridia from human feces in and about the house, especially where sanitary disposal of feces is lacking and where poor hygienic conditions exist. The infection is transmitted by ingestion of embryonated eggs from soil or salads or other foods eaten raw. The disease is communicable as long as mature, fertilized female worms live in the intestine. Each worm produces about 20,000 eggs a day.

Worms mature about 2 mos. after ingestion.

None.

The treatment of choice is Mebendazole (Vermox®), 100 mg b.i.d. for 3 days (regardless of age and weight of patients) or pyrantel pamoate (Antiminth®), 11 mg/kg (max: 1 gm) in 1 dose. The feces of cabinmates should be examined for eggs.

Disease	Incubation Period	Isolation	Prevention and Treatment
Cat Scratch Fever This is a benign infection which develops 3-4 days after a scratch or bite of a cat. A red inflammatory papule first develops resembling a furuncle. Two to 3 weeks later, regional lymph nodes become enlarged, and the overlying skin becomes inflamed. Symptoms of malaise, headache, and fever persist for days or weeks until the suppurating nodes rupture. There is usually quick recovery. The etiologic agent is unknown. The disease is not communicable from man-to-man. Skin test is not commercially available.	7-12 days. (3-30 days)	None.	No specific treatment is available.
Chickenpox (Varicella) This is an acute infectious disease caused by the varicella-zoster virus and is the same agent which is the cause of herpes zoster. The patient will have slight fever and mild constitutional symptoms. The eruption is maculopapular that becomes vesicular for 3-4 days which subsequently leaves scabs. Lesions may be upon the scalp, mucous membranes, and in the respiratory tract. Lesions are usually more abundant on the covered parts of the body. The skin lesions commonly occur in successive crops and are in various stages of maturity. The reservoir of infection is presumably the secretions of the respiratory tract in infected persons. Scabs are not infectious. This is one of the most communicable diseases. It is transmitted from person-to-person by direct contact or droplet infection and indirectly from articles freshly soiled by discharges from the skin and mucous membranes.	10-21 days average 14 days.	This disease is considered communicable 1-2 days before and for 6 days after the appearance of the first vesicles.	There is no specific treatment. The camper should be isolated in the infirmary for 7 days during the period of communicability. Visitors to and from the camp should be discouraged. An experimental vaccine is being tested but is not available at present. Though controversial, children with varicella should probably not receive salicylates because of association with subsequent development of Reye's syndrome.
Herpes Zoster (Shingles) This is thought to be a recurrence of varicella virus that has remained dormant in a nerve ganglion. Pain and itching may precede the nerve involvement with papules and vesicles forming several days later along the dermatome pattern of the nerve. The vesicular fluid is infecti-		Until all lesions have crusted.	As above as this is the same virus.

ous and can produce varicella in susceptible individuals. The trigeminal and intercostal nerves are frequently involved.

Common Cold

This is an acute catarrhal infection of the upper respiratory tract characterized by coryza, lacrimation, irritation of the nasopharynx, chilliness, and malaise lasting 2-7 days. Complications, such as sinusitis, otitis media, laryngitis, tracheitis, and bronchitis are common. Many respiratory viruses may produce this disease. Bacteria (i.e., pneumococci, streptococci, H. influenzae) are thought to play a role in the suppurative complications. The infection is transmitted by direct contact or by droplet infection, and indirectly by handkerchiefs or eating utensils freshly soiled by infected persons.

24 hrs.

The disease is considered communicable 1 day before the onset of symptoms and 5 days thereafter. Isolation is very difficult as most patients do not seek medical advice.

There is no specific treatment, but suppurative complications should be treated with appropriate antibiotics.

Diphtheria

This is an infection caused by the toxin of *Corynebacterium diphtheria* characterized by an acute febrile illness with inflammation of the tonsils, throat, and nose. A one-sided discharge may be a warning of nasal infection. Diphtheria may involve the skin. This appears as localized, punched-out ulcers. The absorption of toxin produces cranial nerve palsies and myocarditis. Fatality is usually 2-4 percent. Diagnosis is made by clinical symptomatology and by bacteriologic examination of discharges and cultures of the nose and throat. The disease is transmitted by contact with infected person or with articles soiled by secretions.

2-6 days.

The patient should be isolated following completion of antibiotic therapy until 2 cultures from the nose and 2 from the throat are negative. All articles containing discharges from the infected person should be incinerated. The disease is considered communicable usually for 2 to 4 wks. in untreated patients or 1-2 days in antibiotic treated patients.

The only effective prevention is through active immunization. If diphtheria is present in the patient, antitoxin should be given before bacteriologic verification (20,000-100,000 units, depending upon the site, severity and duration of the disease). Half may be given intravenously. Neither penicillin nor antitoxin shorten the period of communicability. Vigorous scrubbing of cutaneous diphtheria with soap, water, and antimicrobials are recommended.

Antitoxin is probably of no value for cutaneous lesions, but some give

I.V.—intravenously

DT—pediatric diphtheria tetanus toxoid

Td—adult diphtheria tetanus toxoid

*The possibility of allergic reaction should be kept in mind. (See Chapter X, Anaphylaxis.)

Disease	Incubation Period	Isolation	Prevention and Treatment

(Diphtheria continued)			20,000-40,000 units of antitoxin.
			
			The following is a suggested dosage regimen for passive immunization in pharyngeal and nasal diphtheria (the dosage is purely empiric).
			
			Dosage/Units
			
			Mild nasal or Pharyngeal — Up to 40,000 I.V.
			
			Severe Pharyngeal or laryngeal. Brawny edema or symptoms over 48 hrs. — Up to 100,000 I.V.
			
			Erthromycin (40 mg/kg/day) or procaine penicillin G (300,000 to 600,000 U daily) should be given parenterally for 14 days. Penicillin and erthromycin are *not* a substitute for antitoxin.
			
			All intimate contacts should be (1) cultured and (2) kept under surveillance for 7 days:
			  a. Asymptomatic, previously immunized should receive a DT or Td depending on age.
			  b. Asymptomatic unimmunized or of doubtful immunization should receive:
			    (1) erythromycin (40 mg/kg/day) orally for 7 days or benzathine penicillin (600,00 to 1.2 million U intramuscularly);

(2) a DT or Td depending on age; and
(3) cultures both before and after prophylaxis.

c. Asymptomatic, unimmunized or of doubtful immunization who cannot be kept under surveillance should:

(1) receive benzathine penicillin G (600,00-1.2 million U intramuscularly); and,

(2) an initial dose of DT or TD depending on age.

Enterobiasis vermicularis (pinworm or thread worm)

This is an intestinal round worm which infects only man. Eggs are infective within a few hours after leaving the gastrointestinal tract. After ingestion, the eggs hatch in the stomach and small intestine. The young worms mature in the lower small intestine and large bowel. Gravid worms migrate to the rectum and perianal area where they discharge eggs. Infected individuals complain of itching in the perianal region. The diagnosis may be made by swabbing the perianal area with a Scotch® tape applicator in the morning before defecation and looking for the eggs with the aid of a microscope. The disease is transmitted by infected persons as long as they harbor the worms, and the transfer is by hand from the anal region to the mouth.

2-6 wks.

The treatment of choice is either Mebendazole (Vermox®), 100 mg in 1 dose regardless of age and weight of patients; or Phrantel pamoate (Antiminth®), 11 mg/kg in 1 dose (1 gm max.).

One may treat the contacts. If symptoms reappear, repeat treatment in 2 wks.

Enterovirus Infections

(Coxsackie A and B, ECHO, Poliovirus)

There are over 70 different antigenic types including the above groups. They are more frequently associated with disease in the summer and the fall in the U.S.A.

None.

128/THE CAMP HEALTH MANUAL

Disease	Incubation Period	Isolation	Prevention and Treatment
(Enterovirus Infections continued)			
Coxsackie A There are 23 different antigenic types. The virus is found primarily in the oropharynx and stool and may be excreted in stool as long as 2 weeks or more after infection. Associated with nonspecific febrile illness which may have a macular, maculopapular, or vesicular rash with it, especially in young children. Diseases associated with this group of viruses include acute lymphonodular pharyngitis, herpangina, meningitis, acute respiratory infection, and rarely paralytic disease.	Average 3-5 days (2 days-2 wks.).	Enteric precautions.	Supportive therapy only as there is no specific therapy. No vaccines are available.
Coxsackie B There are 6 different antigenic types. These have been associated with epidemics of pleurodynia (pleuritic pain), non-specific febrile illness with or without macular, maculopapular and uricarial rashes, meningitis, acute respiratory infections, myocarditis and pericarditis in young adults, and rarely paralytic disease.	2-3 days (2 days-2 wks.).	Enteric precautions.	Supportive therapy as there is no specific therapy. No vaccines are available.
ECHO (Enteric Cytopathic Human Orphans) There are 31 antigenically different viruses known presently. These viruses have been associated with non-specific febrile illness with and without rashes, meningitis, meningoencephalitis, and rarely encephalitis or paralysis. These have been reported in epidemics as well as sporadic cases.	3-5 days.	Enteric precautions.	Supportive therapy only as there is no specific treatment. No vaccines are available.
Poliomyelitis There are 3 different poliovirus types (1, 2, 3). These cause non-specific febrile illness but are associated with paralytic disease. Very few paralytic cases are reported in the United States since the introduction of poliovirus vaccines. There is pleocytosis of 50-300 cells predominantly mononuclear. This may be found in any entero-	7-14 days (5-35 days).	Enteric precautions.	Supportive therapy only as there is no specific therapy. There are 2 polio-virus vaccines available: oral live attenuated, and inactivated (killed). Usually 3-4 doses

viral (Coxsackie A, B, ECHO, polio) infection involving the central nervous system.

Food-Borne Diseases
The etiology of food-borne disease in the United States is bacterial in 66 percent, chemical in 24 percent, parasitic in 8 percent and viral in 3 percent. *Salmonella, Staphylococcus, C. perfringens,* and *Shigella* are the principal offenders. Meat and poultry are the most common sources.

A. Botulism
This is a grave, afebrile poisoning characterized by headache, weakness, constipation, and oculomotor or other motor paralysis. Toxins A, B, E, and F are produced by *Clostridium botulinum*. Type A predominated in the western states, Type B in the eastern states and Type E in Alaska. Improperly home-canned food, seafood, fish, and rarely, commercially packaged food are the sources of the toxin. Fatality is 11 percent.

12-48 hrs. (6 hrs.-8 days)

None.

are given to provide adequate protection.

The local health authorities should be notified in any food-borne epidemic at a camp to aid in the control.

Trivalent (ABE) anti-toxin is recommended unless the toxin type is known. Supportive measures will be necessary, and the patient should be transferred to a hospital.

B. Staphylococcal food poisoining
The etiology is the enterotoxin produced by some strains of *Staphylococcus aureus*. There are 5 distinct heat-stable enterotoxins (A, B, C, D, E) with A and D being most common in the U.S.A. The illness is characterized by a sudden onset of vomiting, prostration, and sometimes diarrhea. Previously associated with custard-filled pastries and salads, meats are now more frequently the source with nearly one-third involving ham.

1-7 hrs.

None.

Primarily supportive measures. Prevention is optimum cooking and refrigeration of food, particularly meat and dairy products. There should be a search for contaminated food and an examination of food handlers for pyogenic skin infections.
  The handler with such an infection should be removed from his job.

(Food-Borne Disease continued)

C. Clostrida perfringens food poisoning

The etiology is due to toxins of Type A strains of *Clostridium perfringens*, both heat-resistant and stable. The symptoms are those of an afebrile illness with an acute on set of diarrhea. Meat or poultry are the most common sources and quantitative counts of 100,000 organisms/gm or greater considered compatible with food-borne disease.

Incubation Period	Isolation	Prevention and Treatment
8-24 hrs.	None.	Treatment is primarily supportive. Prevention is accomplished by optimum cooking temperatures and refrigeration to limit proliferation of the organisms.

D. Salmonella

All of the over 2,200 serotypes can cause disease. Almost all outbreaks of salmonella food poisoning can be traced to foods of animal origin; poultry is a common cause of infection. The disease can also be transmitted to man by infected persons or carriers or from infected pets.

Typhoid fever is due to a specific group D salmonella and is infrequently now associated with epidemics.

Incubation Period	Isolation	Prevention and Treatment
6-72 hrs.	Enteric precautions during the acute phase. The communicable period persists as long as organisms are excreted. The currently available typhoid vaccine is not indicated in outbreaks or in summer camps.	Ampicillin, amoxicillin or chloramphenicol are most effective at present. Antibiotics may not alter the intestinal disease and may prolong the carrier state. Therefore, they are not indicated except in patients with chronic intestinal disease or hemoglobinopathies. Chloramphenicol, amoxicillin, or ampicillin are indicated in extraintestinal disease. Trimethoprim-sulfamethoxazole is an alternative therapy when specific drug allergies exist. Appropriate cooking of food and refrigeration aid in prevention of the disease. Careful screening of kitchen personnel, safe water supply, and sanitary disposal of human excretion

APPENDIX I/131

E. Shigella
(See Shigellosis, page 145.)

F. Streptococcal
(See Streptococcal infections, page 145.)

Gonorrhea

This is an infection caused by *Neisseria gonorrheae* and produces a mucopurulent vaginal or urethral discharge in female and urethral discharge in males. Diagnosis is established by bacterial culture. The disease is transmitted from humans by direct contact with infected persons from willing or unwilling sexual contact. Pharyngeal, rectal, as well as urethral and vaginal secretions should be cultured. An attack does not confer immunity.

Complicated gonococcal infections (acute pelvic inflammatory disease, epididymitis, disseminated infection, or ophthalmic infection) should be transferred to a hospital for diagnosis and management.

Incubation: 3–5 days.

Communicability: For 24 hrs. after treatment.

Treatment:
1. Aqueous procaine penicillin—4.8 million units intramuscularly plus 1 gm probenecid by mouth.
2. Ampicillin, 3.5 gm, or amoxicillin, 3.0 gm, plus 1 gm probenecid by mouth.
3. Tetracycline, 0.5 gm 4 times daily for 5 days by mouth (10.0 gm total).
4. If the infection is caused by penicillinase producing gonococci, spectinomycin, 2.0 gm intramuscularly is the drug of choice.

Investigation should be carried out to determine the source (contact).

Hepatitis A (Infectious Hepatitis)

This is an acute infection caused by the hepatitis A virus which may present anorexia, vomiting, fatigue, lassitude, and abdominal discomfort. The liver may be enlarged and tender. Icterus may be present. Many children are anicteric. Liver function tests are abnormal. The source of infection is from man-to-man, primarily by a fecal-oral route via water or food. This virus may be demonstrated by electron microscopy, and methods are aid in the control of this infection.

Incubation: 25–30 days (15–20 days).

Communicability: Most communicable during the wk. prior to and the wk. after onset of jaundice. Patients should be placed on enteric isolation.

Treatment: No specific treatment. Immune globulins (IGs) are recommended for household and other close contacts.

Recommended dosage for post-exposure is 0.02 ml/kg body weight intramuscularly as soon as possible after ex-

Disease	Incubation Period	Isolation	Prevention and Treatment
(Hepatitis A continued) available to demonstrate the antibody. Fatality is about 0.19 percent.			posure. This is effective for about 6 wks.
Hepatitis B (Serum Hepatitis) This acute infection is caused by the hepatitis B virus. There are several different antigens and antibodies of this virus that can be demonstrated by serological tests. This virus is transmitted by infective serum or plasma by inoculation, through minute skin cuts or abrasions, mucosal surfaces, through sexual contact with infected secretions or possibly contact with environmental surfaces or vectors. Clinical disease is insidious in onset with anorexia, malaise, vomiting, abdominal pain, or jaundice.	90 days 2–6 mos.	Only needle and syringe isolation is necessary.	No specific treatment. A new hepatitis B vaccine will soon be available. Hepatitis B immunoglobulin (HBIG) or post-exposure prophylaxis depends on type of exposure and should be given within the first 7 days. The dosage recommendations are:
		Exposure to: (patient's blood, plasma) with	HB_sAG* Testing within 7 days	Recommended Prophylaxis
		HB_sAG* positive	Yes	HBIG (0.06 ml/kg) Immediately and 1 mo. later
		HB_sAG* status unknown Source known: High Risk (homosexual, drug abusers, etc.)		Immune globulin (IG) (0.06 ml/kg) immediately TEST POSITIVE-HBIG (0.06 ml/kg) immediately and 1 mo. later TEST NEGATIVE- Nothing

	Low Risk (young child)		Nothing or IG (0.06 ml/kg)
	HB_sAG^* status unknown Source unknown	No No	Nothing or IG (0.06 ml/kg) *HB_SAG - hepatitis B surface antigen

Non-A—Non-B
There may be several different types of viruses in this group. They are thought to be transmitted primarily by blood. There are no accurate tests for diagnosis. Symptoms are similar to hepatitis due to A or E viruses. The mortality rate is at present unknown. There is an insidious onset of jaundice and the infection appears to run a chronic or remitting course over several weeks.

2-7 wks. are suggested.

As for Hepatitis A and B.

None known. No specific recommendations, but it is reasonable to apply recommendations for Hepatitis B.

Herpangina
This is an acute infection due to Coxsackie Group A viruses with sudden onset of fever and small vesicular lesions of the pharynx which promptly ulcerate. The illness lasts 3-5 days, and there may be recurrence of fever 1 week later. A definite diagnosis can be made by recovery of the virus from the lesion. The demonstration of neutralizing and complement fixing antibody response will confirm the diagnosis. The disease may be confused with herpetic stomatitis. The lesions in the latter are larger and are usually in front of the mouth. The disease is transmitted by direct contact with infected persons and by droplet spread.

3-5 days.

The camper should be isolated in the infirmary for several days.

There is no specific treatment.

Infectious Mononucleosis
The etiologic agent is the Epstein-Barr virus (EBV). The cytomegalovirus (CMV) also produces a similar clinical syndrome in adolescents and young adults. The infection is transmitted from person-to-person. The disease may be manifested by exudative tonsillitis with enlargement of lymph nodes and spleen, or without throat manifesta-

Probably 2-8 wks.

Period of communicability is unknown. The camper should be sent home because of the possible protracted nature of the illness. This decision may be

There is no specific treatment.

Disease	Incubation Period	Isolation	Prevention and Treatment
(Infectious Mononucleosis continued) tions but with fever and lymph node involvement. A rash of variable morphology is an irregular occurrence. Jaundice and meningoencephalitis are sometimes seen. The disease is rarely fatal.		tempered by the severity of the individual case.	
Influenza There are 3 types of viruses: A, B, and C. Types A and B cause recurrent epidemics with antigenically distinct types. The onset is abrupt with fever, chilliness, aches and pain, prostration, coryza, sore throat, and cough. This persists for 1-6 days and is a self-limited disease. Recovery is usual, although bacterial pneumonia may be a complication. Laboratory confirmation of the diagnosis can be achieved by recovery of the virus from throat washings or by demonstration of a significant rise in antibodies against a specific influenza virus in serums obtained during the acute and convalescent phases of the disease. The disease is transmitted by direct contact through droplet infection.	1-3 days.	The disease is considered communicable for approximately 1 wk. after onset, and the patient should be isolated during the acute illness.	Active immunization with currently available vaccines will appreciably reduce the incidence, provided the prevailing strain of virus matches closely the antigenic components of the vaccine used. Duration of protection is uncertain (possibly 1 yr.). The effective approach would be to use the vaccine in advance of an anticipated epidemic. If an epidemic does strike a camp, it may be of interest to identify the virus. Nose and throat cultures and samples of blood sera could be sent to one of many influenza centers. The local health authorities will be of help. There is no specific treatment for all 3 types, though amantidine has been used prophylactically and may have some therapeutic effect on the type A virus.

Leptospirosis
There are over 150 different serotypes, not all of which have been associated with infection in man. The clinical manifestations vary from mild flu-like febrile illness to nephritis, meningitis, hepatitis, pneumonitis, and myocarditis. Symptoms are consistent with those of the organ or organs involved. Conjunctival infection, jaundice, meningismus, headache, and rash, including petechiae and hematuria, are seen. The disease may be mild to severe requiring several weeks of hospitalization. The spirochetes are best isolated from the urine but require special laboratory media. Hemagglutinating and immuno-fluorescent methods are available to demonstrate increases in serum antibodies. The reservoir is the urine of chronically infected animals (cattle, dogs, swine, horses, rats, and other wild rodents) and transmitted to man by contact with the animal, animal carcasses, or wading in infected ponds or streams. It enters through the mucous membrane or broken skin. Man-to-man transmission is doubtful.

2-20 days.

None.
Urine of man may contain organisms for 10-20 days after onset.

Penicillin, streptomycin and tetracyclines are leptospiracidal *in vitro* but are of questionable value for the infection in man unless begun within 2-4 days after onset of illness. The public health authorities should be notified and can help by suggestions for the irradication of rats.

Meningitis (Bacterial)
This is an acute bacterial infection caused most frequently by pneumococci *(Streptococcus pneumoniae)* meningococcus *(Neisseria meningitidis)* or influenza *(Haemophilus influenzae* type B) organisms. Other bacteria rarely cause meningitis in normal individuals. Fever, severe headache, nausea and often vomiting, signs of meningeal irritation and petechial rash (most frequent with meningococcal) are present. Collapse and shock may occur in fulminant meningococcal infection. The period of communicability is for 24 hours after beginning antibiotic therapy. The organisms are isolated from blood or cerebrospinal fluid.

Variable, 1-7 days.

For 24 hrs. after onset of antibiotic administration.

Penicillin or ampicillin and chloramphenicol intravenously are the specific therapeutic agents. This is a medical emergency and patients should be transferred to the hospital immediately. Prophylaxis in meningococcal infection for close contacts is rifampin—adults, 600 mg twice daily; children from 1 mo. to 12 yrs., 10 mg/kg twice daily for 2 days (max: 1,200 mg/day). Meningococcus vaccines are available for groups A, C, Y, and W-135 and may be considered as an adjunct to chemopro-

Disease	Incubation Period	Isolation	Prevention and Treatment
(Meningitis continued)			phylaxis for high risk contact persons. Prophylaxis for H. *influenzae* type B infection is being investigated using rifampin—adults 600 mg daily; children 20 mg/kg daily for 4 days (max: 600 mg/day). There is an experimental H. *influenzae* type B vaccine being investigated.
Mumps (Epidemic Parotitis) This is an acute infection caused by the mumps virus characterized by a sudden onset of fever and swelling and tenderness of one or more of the salivary glands. The parotid glands are most often involved. The ovaries and testicles are more frequently involved in persons beyond puberty. Orchitis and meningoencephalitis may occur without involvement of the salivary glands. The reservoir of infection is in the saliva of infected persons. The mode of transmission of the infection is by droplet spread and by direct contact with the infected person.	16-18 days (12-25 days).	The camper should be isolated until the swelling of the salivary glands subsides. The disease is considered communicable from about 7 days before and for 9 days after onset of symptoms.	There is no specific treatment. A live virus vaccine is available to prevent this disease. Mumps vaccine may be given to all susceptible and unvaccinated individuals. It would be wise to discourage visitors to the camp.
Pediculosis This is an infestation with adult lice, larvae, or nits of the scalp and hairy parts of the body and is caused by *Pediculus humanus*, head louse or body louse, and *Phthirus pubis*, crab louse. The infestation is transmitted by direct contact with an infected person or indirectly with clothing from an infested person.	The eggs hatch in a wk. and reach maturity in 2 wks.	No isolation.	The patients should bathe and scrub thoroughly with soap and water. Then apply 1 ounce of 1 percent gamma benzene hexachloride (Kwell®) shampoo to the scalp thoroughly and leave the shampoo on for 5-10 minutes. After rinsing, comb the hair with a fine tooth comb to remove nits.

Application of a 1:1 solution of white vinegar and water followed by a shower helps dissolve the nits cemented to the hairs. Do not repeat shampoo more than twice in 1 wk.

For body or pubic lice, apply 1 percent gamma benzene hexachloride (Kwell®) cream or lotion to all the skin below the neck and leave for 24 hrs., then rebathe. If eyebrows and eyelashes are involved, ophthalmic grade petrolatum ointment should be applied twice daily for 8-10 days to smother the lice.

Bed clothes, towels, caps, and clothing should be decontaminated by washing in detergent and hot water and drying. Treat contacts prophylactically.

Pertussis (Whooping Cough)
This is an acute bacterial infection caused by *Bordetella pertussis* involving the trachea, bronchi, and bronchioles. The duration of the disease is usually for 1-2 months. There are three stages: catarrhal, paroxysmal, and convalescent. The most characteristic is the paroxysmal stage characterized by repeated series of violent coughs, frequently ending with a crowing type of inspiratory whoop. Case fatality is low and is less than 0.5 percent. The etiologic agent is recovered during the catarrhal and early paroxysmal stages by nasopharyngeal swab. The disease is transmitted by direct contact with infected persons by droplet spread and indirectly by articles freshly soiled with discharges from infected persons.

7-10 days (5-21 days).

The patient should be isolated until the diagnosis is established and then sent home. The disease is considered communicable for 7 days after exposure to 4 wks. after the onset of symptoms.

Erythromycin given for 7-10 days will decrease communicability.

Erthromycin may be given prophylactically for 5-10 days to all contacts, but the data regarding protection is unknown.

Pertussis vaccine boosters should *NOT* be given contacts over 6 yrs. of age.

Disease	Incubation Period	Isolation	Prevention and Treatment
Pneumonia, bacterial This is an acute bacterial infection caused by *Streptococcus pneumoniae*. There are also other etiologic agents, such as *Streptococcus pyogenes* (Group A hemolytic streptococci) and *Hemophilus influenzae* type B and, rarely, *Staphylococcus aureus* and *Enterobacteriaceae*. Sudden onset of chills, fever, pain in chest, productive cough, dyspnea and leucocytosis characterize pneumonia. Roentgenogram may disclose lobar or bronchial distribution of the disease prior to other evidence of consolidation. Fatality has been greatly reduced since the advent of penicillin and other antimicrobial drugs. The disease is transmitted by droplet spread and by clinical contact with patients and carriers, or through articles freshly soiled with discharges from nose and throat of such persons. This disease occurs in association with other infections of the respiratory tract, particularly epidemic influenza. The clinical manifestations may be the same as in lobar pneumonia.	1-3 days.	The patient should be treated in the infirmary. The disease is considered communicable. Penicillin will eliminate the pneumococcus from most patients in 24 hrs.	Penicillin is the specific treatment with erythromycin being the drug of choice for those allergic to penicillin. Contacts require no specific therapy. A pneumococcal vaccine is given to patients with specific diseases (sickle cell anemia, post-splenectomy). Specific antibiotic therapy is available for each organism (group A streptococcus-penicillin; *Hemophilus influenzae* type B - ampicillin, chloramphenicol; *Staphylococcus aureus*-semi-synthetic penicillin).
Pneumonia, Mycoplasma (Primary atypical pneumonia) This is an acute respiratory infection characterized by an insidious onset, chilliness, fever, headache, malaise, and cough. Physical findings in lungs are minimal. Roentgenograms will reveal patchy infiltration. The leukocyte count is normal. The duration of the illness is about 1 week and complications are infrequent. Fatality is about 1 per 1,000. Demonstration of a four-fold or greater titer rise of *Mycoplasma Pneumoniae* confirm the diagnosis in the majority of patients. The etiology is *Mycoplasma pneumoniae*. The disease is transmitted by intimate contact with patients or with articles soiled by secretions from nose and throat of patients. Epidemics have occurred in camps.	7-21 days.	The patient should be treated in the infirmary. The disease is considered communicable during the late incubation period and throughout the febrile illness, but the exact period of communicability is unknown.	Erythromycin until 48 hrs. after defervescence is specific (5-7 days average). Tetracycline is also effective in children over 9 yrs. of age. Overcrowding in cabins should be avoided.

Psittacosis

An acute generalized infection with fever, headache, and early pneumonic involvement, extreme anorexia, prostration, delirium. The etiologic agent is *Chlamydia psittaci*. These agents are antigenically related to lymphogranuloma venerum and trachoma. Laboratory diagnosis is possible during the first week of illness, but is dangerous to laboratory personnel. A rise in titer of complement fixation antibody may be demonstrated in the infected individual. Infected parrots, parakeets, lovebirds, canaries, pigeons, ducks, turkeys, and chickens are reservoirs of infection. Healthy birds occasionally transmit infection through cloacal discharges containing the organism. The infection is transmitted through contact with infected birds, chiefly household pets. The disease is communicable during the acute illness when there is coughing. Birds characteristically have latent infections, but at irregular intervals appear sick and discharge the agent in large quantities. One attack usually confers immunity. All ages are susceptible.

7-14 days.

The camper should be isolated during the acute febrile stage and should be transferred to a hospital. The infirmary room should be cleaned thoroughly after the camper is removed.

The tetracycline antibiotics are felt to be effective if given for 10-21 days. Chloramphenicol is an alternative drug.

Rat Bite Fever

Haverhill fever is caused by the *Streptobacillus moniliformis*. There is usually a history of a rat bite within 10 days. The site of the bite is inflammed, and there is swelling of the regional lymph nodes. The disease is characterized by sharp febrile episodes alternating with afebrile intervals, morbilliform and petechial rash, polyarthritis and leucocystosis. Bacteriologic examination of the primary lesion, lymph nodes, blood, joint fluid, or by the serum test of specific agglutination will help establish the diagnosis. The reservoir of infection is the infected rat and rarely the squirrel or weasel. The disease is transmitted by the bite of an infected rat. Localized epidemics may occur from contaminated food or milk products. The disease is not transmitted from man-to-man.

Soduko is caused by *Spirillum minus* and produces a chancre-like lesion at the site of the bite with the infecting organisms present in the secretions of the nose,

3-10 days.

None.

The disease may be prevented by rat-proofing and reducing rat population. Pasteurization of milk will prevent Haverhill fever.
Penicillin and tetracyclines are useful for treatment and should be continued for 10-14 days.

7-21 days.

None.

Penicillin is effective treatment.
Control of rat population is most important.

Disease	Incubation Period	Isolation	Prevention and Treatment
(Rat Bite Fever continued) mouth, and conjunctivae of the rat. This is not transmitted from man-to-man. False positive syphilitic serology is present.			
Ringworm Ringworm is a general term applied to mycotic infections of keratinized areas of the body (hair, skin, and nails). This is caused by various genera and species of a group of fungi known collectively as dermatophytes.			
A. Ringworm of the scalp (tinea capitis) Ringworm of the scalp (tinea capitis) is an infection which is caused by species of *Microsporum* and *Trichophyton* and begins as a small papule of alopecia. Infected hairs become brittle and break easily. When the lesion becomes boggy and edematous with non-pyogenic material crusted on the surface of the lesion, it is called a kerion. The lesions may fluoresce when looked at under a Wood's light. Microscopic examination of the hair may show spores within the hair. The fungus should be cultured for genus and species identification. Microscopic examination of the hair in sodium hydroxide shows hyphae and spores. The reservoir of infection resides in lesions on infected man and animals (dog, cat, cattle). The spores may be upon barber clippers, toilet articles, or clothing contaminated with infected hair. The disease is transmitted by direct contact with the source of infection. Children before puberty are highly susceptible to *Microsporum* and most adults are resistant. All ages are susceptible to *Trichophyton*, but children are more susceptible. No immunity is developed. Ringworm of the scalp is caused by *Microsporum audouini*, *M. canis*, and *Trichophyton tonsurans*.	2-3 wks.	Head should be covered with cap. Camper should be sent home once diagnosis is made. Isolation would be impractical.	A specific etiology can be determined by culture of several hairs removed from the border of the lesion. There is no specific management of exposed susceptibles. The antibiotic griseofulvin has been shown to be an effective agent in ringworm of the scalp, body, and nails. This drug inhibits growth of *Trichophyton*, *Microsporum*, and *Epidermophyton*, but is not effective against bacteria, yeast, or any of the systemic mycoses. The recommended dose is 10 mg/kg every 24 hrs. of microcrystalline griseofulvin in a single or divided doses. For children of 30-50 lbs., 125-250 mg/24 hrs.; over 50 lbs., 250-500 mg/24 hrs.

APPENDIX I/141

B. Ringworm of the body (tinea corporis)
Ringworm of the body (tinea corporis) is an infection which is caused by the species *Trichophyton rubrum* and *T. mentagrophytes*; or *Epidermophyton floccosum*. The source is from humans and animals transmitted by personal contact.

Variable, from 1-3 wks.	None.

Treatment may extend from 4-8 wks. Ultra-microsizes griseofulvin is used in about 1/2 the dose of microsized griseofulvin. A boiled and washed cotton skull cap should be worn constantly in case of infections with *M. audouini* or *T. tonsuans* to collect broken hairs and scales.

Commonly used topical antifungal agents—1 percent clotrimazole, 1 percent haloprogen, 2 percent micronazole, or 1 percent tolnaftate. Applications should be made to the area 3 times daily. Continue treatment for 10 days after lesions resolve to prevent recurrence.

C. Ringworm of the feet (tinea pedis)
Tinea pedis is due to various species of fungi of the species *Trichophyton*, especially *Trichophyton rubrum* and *T. mentagraphytes*. This is uncommon before puberty and acquired from public areas such as swimming pools, locker rooms, and shower rooms. It results from contact with skin flakes or colonies of fungi in damp areas after consistent trauma to the feet.

Variable, 2-3 wks.	Not practical.

See topical antifungal agents as described above for ringworm of the body. Severe involvement may require microcrystalline grieseofulvin.

D. Ringworm of the nails (tinea unguium)
This is a chronic infection caused by *Epidermophyton floccusum* and various species of *Microsporum* involving one or more nails of the hand or foot. Fingerna ls are less commonly involved than toenails. The nail gradually thickens, becomes discolored and brittle, and an

Unknown.	None.

Treatment is difficult, cure is difficult and relapse is frequent.
Topical treatment rarely cures and microcrystalline

Disease	Incubation Period	Isolation	Prevention and Treatment
(Ringworm continued) accumulation of caseous-appearing material forms beneath the nail. Microscopic examination of the scrapings after treatment with sodium hydroxide shows the segmented branching mycelial threads. Correct identification is made by culture.			grieseofulvin may require 6-12 mos. for treatment.
Rocky Mountain Spotted Fever This disease is caused by *Rickettsia rickettsii* and is characterized by a sudden onset of fever which may persist for 2 weeks, with headache, conjunctival suffusion and a maculopapular rash. The rash appears on the extremities about the third day and spreads rapidly to most of the body including the palms and soles before becoming petechial. Death is uncommon when treatment is prompt but is still 5-7 percent. The Weil-Felix reaction with Proteus OX-19 and OX-2 becomes positive after 1-12 days. Complement fixation using specific rickettsial antigen and immunoflurorescent tests becomes positive after the Weil-Felix reaction. In the eastern and southern United States, the common vector is the dog tick. *Dermacentor variabilis*, and in the northwestern United States it is the wood tick, *Dermacentor andersoni*. In the southwestern U.S., it is the lone star tick, *Amblyomma americanum*. The infection is passed from generation to generation in ticks and probably is maintained by infected and noninfected larvae feeding upon susceptible wild rodents. The infection is transmitted by the bite of an infected tick. Contamination of the skin with crushed, infected tick tissues or feces may also produce the infection in man. The infection is not communicable from man-to-man. The infection is most prevalent in the Middle Atlantic states, and infection rates are related to chances for contact with infected ticks.	4-8 days (3-12 days).	None.	The infection may be prevented by avoiding tick-infested areas. Careful removal of ticks without crushing and protecting the hands while removing the ticks will also help. Tetracycline or chloramphenicol daily until the patient is afebrile for 2-3 days are effective drugs in the treatment of the infection. The patient is usually ill enough so that hospitalization is necessary and then should be sent home. Active immunization is recommended only for workers exposed to high occupational risk.

Rubella (German Measles)
Rubella is a mild febrile infection caused by a virus with a rash resembling measles and sometimes that of scarlet fever. There are few constitutional symptoms. There is enlargement of the postauricular, suboccipital, or postcervical group of lymph nodes.
   Mild catarrhal symptoms may be present. Absence of Koplik's spots helps distinguish this from measles. Leucopenia is usual during fever.

14-21 days, usually 16 days.

The camper should be in the infirmary for the duration of the illness and 5 days thereafter. The disease is considered communicable from 7 days before until 5 days after the onset of symptoms.

The disease is not a serious one but will disrupt the functioning of the camp, and it is for this reason that isolation measures should be instituted to help prevent the spread of infection. The greatest hazard of the disease is in the possibility of producing congenital malformations if a woman develops the disease during the first trimester of pregnancy.
   A live virus vaccine is available to prevent this disease.

Rubeola (Measles)
Acute, highly communicable viral disease. The prodromal state is characterized by catarrh and Koplik spots upon the buccal mucosa. A morbilliform rash appears upon the third or fourth day, affecting face, body, and extremities, in that order. Leucopenia is usual. The virus is transmitted by air, droplet spread, or direct contact with the infected person and is highly communicable.

10-12 days.

The disease is considered communicable for 5 days before and 4-5 days after the rash appears. The camper should be in the infirmary for the duration of the illness.

There is no specific treatment.
   Complications should be treated with antibiotics. In a camp situation, it would be wise to give gamma globulin to all intimately exposed individuals who have not had the disease and to all susceptible individuals (those who have not been actively immunized).
For protection:
   Dose of gamma globulin is 0.1 ml per lb. of body weight.
   A daily check should be made upon all intimately exposed individuals. Isolation is advisable for all campers

Disease	Incubation Period	Isolation	Prevention and Treatment
(Rubeola continued)			who are running fever until there is demonstration that it is not measles. It is advisable to notify the local health authorities. A live virus vaccine is available to prevent this disease. An effort is being made to eradicate this disease from the U.S.
Scabies This is an infection of the skin caused by the itch mite, *Sarcoptes scabiei*, and is characterized by itching. Burrows appear as slightly grayish-white lines which house the mite and eggs. There may also be papules and vesicles. These usually become pustular due to secondary infection caused by scratching. Lesions are most prominent in the folds of the skin such as finger webs, elbow creases, armpits, between thighs, and under breasts of women. The itch mite is identified by hand lens in scrapings from the burrows. The eggs can be seen microscopically. The disease is transmitted by the transfer of young female mite by direct contact with the skin of infected persons.	Primary infection 2-6 wks. resulting in sensitization. Reinfection symptoms appear within a few days.	None.	The treatment consists of bathing and applying 1 percent gamma benzene hexachloride (Kwell®) or N-ethyl-o-crotonotoluide (Eurax®) to the body from the neck down. The ointment or lotion is left on for 24 hrs. Freshly laundered clothes are put on in the morning. All soiled clothes and bedding should be laundered. Treatment may be repeated in 1 wk. if necessary. The cabinmates may become infected and should be followed closely.

Shigellosis (Bacillary Dysentery)
This is an acute bacterial infection manifested by diarrhea, fever, tenesmus, and sometimes blood and mucus in the stools.

Species of the genus *Shigella sonnei* (dysentery bacilli), *S. flexneri* in the United States are the etiologic agents, and the diagnosis is made by bacteriologic isolation of bacilli from stool. This is transmitted by hand-to-mouth transfer of contaminated material from patients, carriers, food, milk, or water.

1-7 days. Average 2-4 days.

The disease is communicable during the acute infection and until bacteria are absent from the stool, which is rarely longer than 4 weeks. An individual should be isolated, and the feces should be disposed in sanitary fashion. In modern sewage disposal systems feces may be disposed of directly into the sewer without preliminary disinfection. Hand washing is most important in control.

Ampicillin, trimethoprinsulfa are the primary therapeutic agents with tetracycline also of value. Contacts should have stool cultures, and food handlers should be shown to be free of organisms. The food and water should be checked, and the local health authorities should be called in for guidance.

Streptococcal Infections

A. Tonsillitis and pharyngitis
This is an infection caused by *Streptococcus pyogenes*. There are over 60 serologically distinct types of Group A streptococci. The infection is characterized by fever, nausea, vomiting, sore throat, exudative tonsillitis or pharyngitis, tender cervical adenopathy, leucocytosis, enanthem (strawberry tongue), and rash (exanthem). The rash will appear if the infected organism is an erythrogenic toxin producer and the patient has no antitoxin immunity. Injection and edema of the pharynx involve the faucial pillars and soft palate and often the hard palate. Petechiae are sometimes present. The rash is a fine erythema, punctate, blanching upon pressure and is most often upon the chest and folds of the thighs. The desquamation during convalescence is seen at the tips of the fingers and toes. The nonsuppurative sequelae which are most important are glomerulonephritis and rheumatic fever. There is good evidence that adequate treatment

2-5 days.

The patient should be isolated for at least 1 day after starting therapy with penicillin. The disease is considered communicable during the incubation and clinical illness. A carrier state may persist for months. Adequate treatment of the acutely ill patient and carrier with penicillin will eliminate probability of transmission in about 2 days.

Most state laboratories are now organized to identify Group A hemolytic streptococci. The absence of rash does not decrease the danger of streptococcal infection. Cabinmates and other close contacts should have throat cultures. The entire kitchen staff should have throat cultures. The specific treatment is the administration of:
1. Benzathine penicillin I.M. 600,000 units for those weighing less than 60 lbs. and 1,200,000 units for those over 60 lbs.

Disease	Incubation Period	Isolation	Prevention and Treatment
(Streptococcal Infections continued) of the infection will appreciably lower the possibility of developing rheumatic fever. Streptococcal sore throat is scarlet fever without a rash. The manifestations are the same as described above except the toxic manifestations, rash, and desquamation do not occur. The laboratory can aid by demonstrating a typable Group A streptococcus on the throat culture, antihyaluronicIase, and a rise in serum antibody titer of antistreptolysin O or antideoxyribonuclease B (DNAse B) from acute to the convalescent phase of the illness. Antibacterial immunity develops only against the type of Group A streptococcal which caused the illness and lasts several years. Several attacks of streptococcal sore throat due to a different type of streptococcus are not uncommon. Immunity against erythrogenic toxin and rash develops within a week after onset of the disease, and second attacks of scarlet fever are uncommon.			2. Oral penicillin 200,000-250,000 units T.I.D. or Q.I.D. for 10 days. 3. Erythromycin or cephalexin may be given for 10 days for those allergic to penicillin.
B. Erysipelas Erysipelas is an acute infection characterized by fever, constitutional symptoms, leucocytosis, and a red, tender edematous spreading lesion of the skin with a definite raised border. Group A streptococci may be isolated from the margin of the skin lesion, nose and throat, and occasionally from the blood. This infection is rarely encountered in summer camps, but if it is, the management is the same as that noted under therapy for tonsillitis and pharyngitis. The infection is transmitted by direct contact with a patient or carrier or by indirect contact through objects handled or by droplet spread.	See above.	See above.	See above.
C. Streptococcal infections have resulted in explosive outbreaks of infection following the ingestion of contaminated milk or other food.			

Tuberculosis

This is a chronic bacterial disease caused by *Mycobacterium tuberculosis*. The human type causes nearly all the pulmonary tuberculosis. Primary infection usually goes unnoticed clinically. Some patients have fever, vague constitutional symptoms, or roentgenographic evidence of infiltration of the lungs or enlarged tracheobronchial nodes. Pleurisy with effusion may occur. Disseminated disease is more likely within the first 6-12 months. Usually the lesions heal spontaneously, and calcification of the pulmonary or tracheobronchial nodes may follow. Active pulmonary involvement has a variable course, and the symptomatology and signs will be determined by the extent of involvement. Specific diagnosis is by demonstration of tubercle bacilli in sputum by smear and by recovery of the organism by culture. Gastric washings may be examined where sputum is difficult to obtain. The tuberculin test is positive in active tuberculosis except in critically ill persons. Extrapulmonary tuberculosis is an early or late result of hematogenous dissemination of organisms during the primary phase.

Respiratory secretions of persons with "open" (bacillary-positive) pulmonary tuberculosis are the source of infection. The mode of transmission is by the coughing and sneezing of patients with open pulmonary tuberculosis. Infection usually results from continued and intimate exposure. Susceptibility is general.

In most Western nations the prevalence and mortality are declining. Mortality rates commonly reflect the social and economic welfare of a region.

Primary lesions, 4-6 wks.

A person can transmit the infection as long as tubercle bacilli are being discharged. Degree of communicability depends upon number of bacilli discharged. If a camper is suspected of having tuberculosis, he should be sent home and should be isolated. If one of the camping personnel develops evidence of tuberculosis, initial isolation is indicated and subsequently he/she should be transferred to a hospital. Parents of campers should be notified so that there is adequate followup after the camping season. If anyone at camp should develop tuberculosis, the public health authorities should be notified. Those in close contact with the patient should be skin-tested except known positive reactors. They should get a chest roentgenogram. All new skin test converters should get a chest roentgenogram.

The standard tuberculin test consists of Purified Protein Derivative containing Tween as a stabilizer (PPDS) containing 5 tuberculin units (TU) in 0.1 ml. This quantity is given intradermally on the volar surface of the forearm and read at 48 hrs. The area of induration is recorded. Induration of more than 10 mm. is positive. Lesions less than 10 mm. are indeterminate. Skin sensitivity develops 2-10 wks. after infection.

Specific Treatment:
Tuberculin convertors.
Prophylaxis is given to all patients under 35 yrs. of age whose tuberculin skin test converts from negative to positive. Adults—Isoniazid, 300 mg daily;
Pyridozine—15-50 mg daily. Children—Isoniazid, 10 mg/kg/daily (max: 300 mg); Pyridozine, 15-50 mg daily for children over 11 yrs. of age—treat 12 mos.
Pulmonary tuberculosis: Adults—Isoniazid, 300 mg daily. Rifamphin, 600 mg daily; Pyridozine, 15-50 mg daily. Children—Isoniazid, 10-20 mg/kg/day (max: 300 mg); Rifampin, 10-20 mg/kg/day (max. 600 mg daily); Pyridoxine, 15-50 mg over

Disease	Incubation Period	Isolation	Prevention and Treatment
(Tuberculosis continued)			11 yrs. of age—for 9-12 mos. Miliary tuberculosis and tuberculous meningitis—3 drugs: Isoniazid and Rifampin in the dosage prescribed for pulmonary tuberculosis, and Ethambutol, adults and children, 15 mg/kg/day (max: 1,500 mg). Should not be used in children too young to test color vision. Streptomycin, adults and children, 15 mg/kg/day (max: 1 gm)—18-24 mos. duration.
Tularemia This is an infectious disease of wild animals and man caused by *Francisella tularensis*. The onset is marked by chills, fever, and prostration. Lymph nodes draining the site of inoculation become swollen and tender. Diagnosis is confirmed by inoculation of animals with material from the local lesions, sputum, or blood, but this is hazardous in the hospital laboratory. Serum bacterial agglutination titers becomes elevated in the 2nd week of infection. Cross-agglutination may occur to brucella antigen. The reservoir of infection may be found primarily in the wild rabbit and hare, woodchuck, and muskrat, though over 100 species of wild mammals, birds, fish, 9 domestic animals and amphibians have all been found infected. The disease is transmitted by the bite of infected flies or ticks and by inoculation of the skin through handling infected animals as in skinning and dressing.	3 days (1-14 days).	None.	The use of rubber gloves by persons engaged in dressing wild game will help prevent the infection, as well as the thorough cooking of meat of wild animals. The drinking of raw water in an area where the disease is prevalent should be avoided. Treatment: Streptomycin for 7-10 days is the usual therapy. Tetracycline and chloramphenicol are less effective and are more likely to result in relapse. A camper will have to be sent to a hospital for diagnosis and will

The ingestion of insufficiently cooked rabbit meat and the drinking of contaminated water are also possible modes of contracting the disease. The disease is not communicable from man-to-man, and the infectious agent may be found in the blood of man during the first 2 weeks of the disease. Refrigerated rabbits kept frozen may be infectious for as long as 3 years.

subsequently have to be sent home.

APPENDIX II

Drugs and Their Dosages

The following are the abbreviations used in this appendix:

- IM   intramuscular
- IV   intravenous
- O   oral
- R   rectal
- SC   subcutaneous
- T   topical
- h   hours

ANALGESICS, NARCOTICS, ANTIPYRETICS, AND STIMULANTS

Acetaminophen
(N-acetyl-p-aminophenol)
(Tempra®, Tylenol®)

Tempra® —4-8 yrs: 120-240 mg
          8-12 yrs: 240 mg
Tylenol® —8-12 yrs: 150-325 mg
          Adult: 1-2 tablets, 4-6 doses (O)

Tempra® —Syrup: 120 mg/5 ml
Tylenol® —Tablets, chewable: 80 mg
          Elixir: 160 mg/5 ml
          Tablets: 325 mg

Acetylsalicylic acid
(Aspirin)

65 mg/kg/24 h
4-6 doses (O, R)

Tablets: 30, 60, 75, 400 mg
(1/2, 1, 1-1/4, 5 grains)

Amphetamine sulfate
(Benzedrine®)

7.5-25 mg/24 h
Divide into 3 doses or as Spansule®
in single dose (O)

Tablets: 5, 10 mg
Spansules: 5, 10, 15 mg

Codeine

For pain: 3 mg/kg/24 h
Divide into 6 doses (O, SC)
For cough: 1/3-1/2 above dose

Cough syrup often contains 10 mg/5 ml

Darvon®
(dextro-propoxyphene hydrochloride)

3 mg/kg/24 h
Divide into 4-6 doses (O)

Capsules: 32, 65 mg

Demerol®
(meperidine hydrochloride)

6 mg/kg/24 h
Max: 100 mg
Divide into 6 doses/24 h
(O, IM, SC)

Tablets: 50, 100 mg
Syrup: 50 mg/5 ml
Ampules or Vials: 25, 50, 75, 100 mg/ml

Dexedrine® sulfate
(dextro-amphetamine sulfate)

7.5-15 mg/24 h
Divide into 3 doses/24 h or as
delayed action in single dose (O)

Tablets: 5 mg
Spansules: 5, 10, 15 mg
Elixir: 5 mg/5 ml

Epinephrine hydrochloride
(Adrenalin® chloride)

Asthma:
  1:1,000 aqueous
  0.01 ml/kg/dose
Repeat every 15-30 min for 2-3 doses (SC)
Max: 0.4 ml/dose
Sus-Phrine® 1:200 dilution in
thioglycollate suspension
0.005 ml/kg/dose (SC)
Max: 0.3 ml/dose. May repeat after 4 h

1:1,000 aqueous:
  Ampules: 1 ml
  Vials: 30 ml

Ampules: 0.5 ml
Vials: 5 ml

Drug	Dosage	Supply
Ephedrine sulfate	3 mg/kg/24 h Max: 30 mg/dose Divide into 4-6 doses/24 h (O, SC, IV)	Capsules: 25, 50 mg Tablets: 25, 50 mg Syrup: 15 mg/4 ml Ampules: 25, 50 mg/ml

Isoproterenol hydrochloride
(Isuprel®)
	For Shock:
	IV Infusion: 5 ug/min
	  Use solution of 1 mg in 200 ml of 5 percent dextrose (1 ml = 5 ug)
	  Administer at rate of 1 ml (5 ug) per min. Monitor blood pressure every 2-3 min
	SC: Initial dose: 0.14 mg
	  range: 0.14-0.2 mg
	IM: Initial dose: 0.2 mg
	  range: 0.02-1 mg
	For Cardiac Standstill and Arrhythmia: (Adult)
	IV: Single dose: 0.02 mg
	  range: 0.01 mg-0.2 mg
		Ampules: (1:5,000)
		1 ml (0.2 mg)—boxes of 5
		5 ml (1 mg)—boxes of 10

Levarterenol bitartrate (Levophed®, norepinephrine)	1.0 ml of 0.2 percent solution (0.1 percent base) in 250 ml diluent. Drip at 0.5 ml/min to give 2 ug/min. Titrate dose with blood pressure. Caution: Slough results from extravascular leakage.	4 ml ampules: (0.2 percent) (1 mg/ml)
Metaraminol bitartrate (Aramine®)	IM or SC. 2-10 mg (0.2-1 ml) IV: 15-100 mg (1.5-10 ml) in 500 ml of isotonic saline solution or 5 percent dextrose solution Titrate speed of infusion by monitoring blood pressure every 2-3 min Direct IV: Single dose: 0.5-5 mg (0.05-0.5 ml for grave emergencies)	1 ml ampules: (10 mg of Aramine® per ml) Also 10 ml vials

APPENDIX II/153

ANALGESICS, NARCOTICS, ANTIPYRETICS, AND STIMULANTS *(continued)*

Morphine sulfate (paregoric contains 0.4 mg of morphine/ml	Preoperative and analgesic 0.1 mg-0.2 mg/kg/dose (SC) Max: 15 mg	Ampules: 8, 10, 15 mg/1 ml Tablets: 10, 15, 20 mg
Theophylline preparations		
Aminophylline (theophylline with ethylenediamine)	15-30 mg/kg/24 h Divide into 4 doses (IV, IM)	IV: 10 ml ampules: 0.25 gm 20 ml ampules: 0.5 gm IM: 2 ml ampules: 0.5 gm
(a) Long-acting (Theo-Dur®)	Under 9 yrs: 100 mg q 12 h (O) 9-12 yrs: 150 mg q 12 h (O) 12-16 yrs: 200 mg q 12 h (O)	Tablets: 100, 200, 300 mg
Gyrocaps® (Slo-Phyllin)	Children: 3-5 mg/kg q 8 h (O) Adult: 4-8 mg/kg q 8 h (O)	Capsules (timed release) 65, 125, 250 mg
(b) Short-acting (Theolair®)	Children: 100 mg q 6 h (O) Adult: 200-250 mg q 6 h (O)	Tablets: 250 mg

ANTIHISTAMINICS

Benadryl® (diphenhydramine hydrochloride)	5 mg/kg/24 h Not to exceed 150 mg/day Divide into 4 doses (O or IM)	Capsules: 25 and 50 mg Tablets (Enteric): 50 mg Elixir: 10 mg/4 ml Ampules: 50 mg/ml Vials: 50 mg/ml
Chlor-Trimeton® (chlorprophenpyridamine maleate and pseudoephedrine sulfate)	Syrup: Adult—4 mg q 6 h Children (5-11 yrs)—2 mg q 6 h Tablets: Same as syrup Repetabs: Adult—8 mg q 8-12 h	Tablets: 4 mg (O) Repetabs®: 8 and 12 mg (O) Syrup: 2 mg/5 ml (O) Injection: 1 ml ampules (10 mg/ml) (IV, IM, SC) 2 ml ampules (100 mg/ml) (IM)

Drug	Dosage	Formulation

Dimetapp®	Adults and Children over 12 yrs
	1 tablet q 12 h (O)
	
	Children (4-12 yrs)
	Elixir: 5-10 ml q 6-8 h (O)
		Extentabs: Brompheneramine maleate 12 mg
		  Phenylephrine HCL 15 mg
		  Phenylpropanolamine HCL 15 mg
		Elixir: Brompheneramine maleate 4 mg
		  Phenylephrine HCL 5 mg
		  Phenylpropanolamine HCL 5 mg

Extendryl®	Adult: 1 SR. cap q 12 h (O)
	  Syrup—10 ml q 4 h (O)
	
	Children (6-12 yrs):
	  1 JR. cap q 12 h (O)
	  Syrup—5 ml q 4 h (O)
	Do not exceed 4 doses/24 h
		Capsules: SR Phenylephrine HCL 20 mg
		  Methscopolomine nitrate 2.5 mg
		  Chlorpheniramine maleate 8 mg
		JR. (1/2 strength of SR.):
		Syrup: Phenylephrine HCL 10 mg
		  Methscopolomine nitrate 1.25 mg
		  Chlorpheniramine maleate 2 mg

PBZ (Formerly Pyribenzamine®)
(tripelennamine hydrochloride)
	Adult: 25-50 mg q 4-6 h (O)
	  Max: 600 mg/24 h
	Children: 5 mg/kg/24 h (O)
	  Max: 300 mg/24 h
	Divide into 4-6 doses/24 h
		Plain tablet (scored): 50 mg
		Coated tablet: 25 mg
		Delayed-action tablets: 50 and 100 mg
		Elixir: 25 mg/5 ml
		Ampules: 25 mg/ml

Periactin®
(cyproheptadine HCL, MSD)
	Adult: 4 mg—2-3 tab/24 h (O)
	  Max: 0.5 mg/kg/24 h
	Children (7-14 yrs):
	  4 mg—2-3 tab/24 h (O)
	  Max: 0.25 mg/kg/24 h
		Tablets: 4 mg

Phenergan® hydrochloride
(Promethazine hydrochloride)
Antihistaminic:
	0.5 mg/kg/dose (O, R, or IM)
	Adult: 25 mg
	Children: 12.5-25 mg
	Antihistaminic:
	  Full dose at night, 1/4 dose AM or prn
	Nausea and vomiting:
	  1/2 to full dose every 4-6 h
	Preoperative: Full or double dose
	Motion sickness:
	  Full dose, repeat 12 h prn
		Tablets (scored): 12.5 and 25 mg
		Suppositories: 25 mg
		Syrup: 6.25 mg/5 ml
		Injection: 25 mg/ml

Teldrin® (chlorpheneramine maleate)	1 Capsule every 12 h (O)	Tablets: 8, 12 mg

SEDATIVES, ANTICONVULSANTS, AND ANTIANXIETY

Drug	Dosage	Forms
Amobarbital sodium (Amytal®)	Same as pentobarbital	Ampules: 65, 125, 250, and 500 mg
Atarax® (hydroxyzine HCL)	Children over 6 yrs: 50-100 mg/24 h in 3 divided doses (O) Adult: 25 mg 3-4 times daily (O)	Tablets: 10, 25, 50, and 100 mg Syrup: 10 mg
Chloral hydrate	50 mg/kg/24 h Not to exceed 1 gm/dose Divide into 3-4 doses (O or R)	Oral use: In solution Rectal use: In cottonseed oil
Dilantin® (diphenylhydantoin sodium)	Children: 4-8 mg/kg/24 h Adult: 300-400 mg/24 h (O) Divide into 3 doses (O or IM)	Tablets: 50 mg Capsules: 30 and 100 mg Suspensions: 100 mg/5 ml Vials: 50 mg/ml
Meprobamate (Miltown®, Equanil®)	25 mg/kg/24 h Children (6-12 yrs): 200-600 mg/24 h Adult: 1,200-1,600 mg/24 h Divide into 2-3 doses/24 h (O)	Tablet: 200 and 400 mg Suspension: 200 mg/5 ml
Paraldehyde	0.15 ml/kg/dose Adult: 4-8 ml (O) (O, R, IM or IV slowly)	USP (liquid)
Pentobarbital sodium (Nembutal®)	Sedation: 1-2 mg/kg/24 h Divide into 3 doses (O, IM, R)	Capsules: 30, 50 and 100 mg Suppositories: 30, 60, 120 and 200 mg Elixirs: 20 mg/4 ml Ampules: 50 mg/ml Vials: 50 mg/ml
Phenobarbital (Luminol®)	Sedation: 2-3 mg/kg/24 h Divide into 3 doses (O, R, or IM) Anticonvulsant: 3-5 mg/kg/dose (IM) Max dose: 300 mg	Tablets: 15, 30, and 100 mg Spansules: 60 and 100 mg Elixir: 20 mg/5 ml Ampules: 130 mg/1 ml

Drug	Dosage	Supply
Secobarbital (Seconal®)	Same as pentobarbital	Tablets (coated): 60 and 100 mg Capsules: 50 and 100 mg Suppositories: 30, 60, 120, and 200 mg Elixir: 22 mg/5 ml Injection: 50 mg/ml
Vistaril® (hydroxyzine pamoate)	Children over 6 yrs: 50-100 mg/24 h in 3-4 divided doses Adult: 25 mg 3-4 times/24 h	Capsules: 25, 50, and 100 mg Oral Suspension: 25 mg/5 ml Vial: 10 ml (25 mg/ml) 1-2 ml Isojet 50 mg/ml

CHEMOTHERAPEUTIC DRUGS

Drug	Dosage	Supply
Amikacin (Amikin®)	15-22 mg/kg/24 h (IM) Max: 0.75-1.0 gm/24 h (IM) Give in divided doses q 8 h	Vials: 0.1, 0.5, 1.0 gm
Amoxicillin trihydrate (Amoxil®, Larotid®, Polymax®, Robamox®, Trimox®, Utimox®, Wymox®)	30-40 mg/kg/day in divided doses q 8 h (O) Max: 2-3 gm/24 h (O)	Capsules: 250, 500 mg Suspension: 125, 250 mg/5 ml Drops: 50 mg/ml
Ampicillin® and Ampicillin Trihydrate	50-100 mg/kg/day in divided doses q 6 h (O) Max: 2-3 gm/24 h (O)	Capsules: 250, 500 mg Suspension: 125, 250, 500 mg/5 ml Chewable Tablets: 125 mg Drops: 100 mg/ml
Ampicillin®, sodium (Amcil®, Omnipen®, Pfizerpan-A®, Pensyn®, Polycillin®, Principen®, SK-Ampicillin®, Supen®, Totacillin®)	100-200 mg/kg/day q 4-6 h in divided doses (IM, IV) Max: 8-10 gm/24 h (IV)	Vials: 0.125, 0.25, 0.5, 1, 2, 4 gm
Bacitracin® ointment	Ointment—apply topically q 6 h	500 units/gm 1.5, 3, 3.75, and 12 gm
Betadine® (providone-iodine)	Cleanse injured area	30 gm tube, 1 lb jar

CHEMOTHERAPEUTIC DRUGS (continued)

Drug	Dosage	Supply
Carbenicillin, disodium (Geopen®, Pyopen®)	400-600 mg/kg/24 h in divided doses q 4-6 h (IM or IV) Max: 30-40 gm/24 h (IV)	Vial: 1, 2, 5, 10 gm
Carbenicillin, idanyl sodium (Geocillin®)	30-50 mg/kg/24 h in divided doses q 6 h (O) Max: 2-3 gm/24 h (O)	Tablets: 382 mg
Cefaclor (Ceclor®)	40 mg/kg/24 h q 8 h in divided doses (O) Max: 1-2 gm/24 h (O)	Capsules: 250, 500 mg Suspension: 125, 250 mg/5 ml
Cefadroxil, monohydrate (Duricef®, Vitracef®)	30 mg/kg/24 h q 12 h in divided doses (O) Adult: 1 gm/24 h (O)	Capsules: 500 mg Suspension: 125, 250, 500 mg/ml
Cefotaxime (Claforan®)	Adult dose: 1 gm q 6-8 h (IM or IV) Max: 12 gm/24 h (IV)	Vials: 0.5, 1, 2 gm
Cephalexin, monohydrate (Keflex®)	25-50 mg/kg/24 h q 6 h in divided doses (O) Max: 2-3 gm/24 h (O)	Capsules: 0.25, 0.5, 1 gm Drops: 100 mg/ml Suspension: 125, 250 mg/5 ml
Cephalothin, sodium (Keflin®)	75-125 mg/kg/24 h q 6 h in divided doses (IM, IV) Max: 8-10 gm/24 h (IV)	Vial: 1, 2, 4 gm
Cephapirin, sodium (Cefadyl®)	40-80 mg/kg/24 h in divided doses q 6 h (IM, IV) Max: 4-6 gm/24 h (IV)	Vial: 1, 2, 4 gm
Chloramphenicol Chloramphenicol palmitate	50-100 mg/kg/24 h q 6 h in divided doses (O) Max: 2-3 gm/24 h (O)	Capsules: 250 mg Suspension: 150 mg/5 ml
Chloramphenicol sodium succinate (Chloromycetin®)	50-100 mg/kg/24 h q 6 h in divided doses (IV) Max: 4-6 gm/24 h (IV) (Blood levels should be checked for appropriate management)	Vial: 1 gm

Clindamycin HCL hydrate	10-25 mg/kg/24 h q 6 h in divided doses (O) Max: 1-2 gm/24 h (O)	Capsules: 75, 150 mg
Clindamycin palmitate HCL	10-25 mg/kg/24 h q 6 h in divided doses (O)	Solution: 75 mg/5 ml
Clindamycin phosphate (Cleocin®)	25-40 mg/kg/24 h q 6 h in divided doses (IM, IV) Max: 2-4 gm/24 h (IV)	Ampules: 0.15, 0.3, 0.6 gm
Demeclocycline HCL (Declomycin®)	10 mg/kg/24 h q 6 h in divided doses (O) Adult: 150 mg q 6 h (O)	Capsules: 150 mg Tablets: 75, 150, 300 mg
Dicloxacillin monohydrate sodium (Dynapen®, Pathocil®)	10-25 mg/kg/24 h q 6 h in divided doses (O) Max: 1-2 gm/24 h (O)	Capsules: 125, 250, 500 mg Suspension: 62.5 mg/5 ml
Doxycycline calcium	5 mg/kg/24 h q 12 h in divided doses (O)	Syrup: 50 mg/5 ml
Doxycycline monohydrate	5 mg/kg/24 h q 12 h in divided doses (O)	Suspension: 25 mg/5 ml
Doxycycline hydrate (Vibramycin®)	5 mg/kg/24 h q 12 h in divided doses (O) Adult: 100 mg q 12 h (O) 5 mg/kg/24 h for 1 day (2-4 h infusion)	Capsules: 50, 100 mg Tablets: 100 mg Vial: 100, 200 mg
Erythromycin (E-Mycin®, Erythromycin®, Filmtab®, Ilotycin®, Pediamycin®, Robimycin®)	40 mg/kg/24 h q 6 h in divided doses (O) Max: 1-2 gm/24 h (O)	Tablets: 250 mg
Erythromycin estolate (Ilosone®)	20-40 mg/kg/24 h q 6-12 h in divided doses (O)	Tablets: 125, 250, and 500 mg Tablets (chewable): 125, 250 mg Drops: 100 mg/ml Suspension: 125, 250 mg/5 ml
Erythromycin ethyl succinate (E.E.S.®, E-Mycin®, Pediamycin®, Wyamycin®)	40 mg/kg/24 h q 6 h in divided doses (O) Max: 1-2 gm/24 h (O)	Tablets: 400 mg Tablets (chewable): 200 mg Drops: 100 mg/2.5 ml Suspension: 200, 400 mg/5 ml

APPENDIX II/159

CHEMOTHERAPEUTIC DRUGS (continued)

Drug	Dose	Form
Erythromycin ethylsuccinate and sulfisoxazole acetyl combination (Pediazole®)	Erythromycin 40-50 mg/kg/24 h and Sulfisoxazole 150 mg/kg/24 h q 6-8 h in divided doses (C) Max: 10 ml q 6 h (O)	Suspension: 200 mg erythromycin 600 mg sulfisoxazole/5 ml
Erthromycin stearate (Bristomycin®, Erythrocin stearate®, Erythromycin stearate®, Ethril®, Pfizer-E®, SK-erythromycin®)	20-40 mg/kg/24 h q 6 h in divided doses (O) Adult: 250 mg q 6 h (O)	Tablets: 125, 250, 500 mg
Gentimicin sulfate (Garamycin®, Garamycin Intrathecal®, U-Gencin®)	3-7.5 mg/kg/24 h q 8 h in divided doses (IM, IV) Max: 300 mg/24 h (IM, IV)	Vial: 20, 80 mg
Griseofulvin (Fulvicin P/G®, Fulvicin U/F®, Grifulvin V®, Grisactin Ultra®, Gris-Peg®)	Ultramicrosize: 5 mg/kg/24 h (O) Microsize: 11 mg/kg/24 h (O) Max: over 50 lbs Ultramicrosize: 125-250 mg/24 h Microsize: 250-500 mg/24 h	Tablets (microsize): 200, 500 mg Tablets (ultramicrosize): 125, 250 mg Suspension: 125 mg/5 ml
Lotrimin® (Clotrimazole)	Apply 3 times a day to affected area	1 percent solution: 10, 20 ml
Mebendazole (Vermox®)	1 dose (100 mg) for pinworms; q 6-12 h x 3 days for other nematodes (O)	Tablets (chewable): 100 mg
Methacycline (Rondomycin®)	10 mg/kg/24 h q 6-12 h in divided doses (O) Adult: 600 mg/24 h (O)	Capsules: 150, 300 mg
Methenamine mandelate (Mandelamine®, Thiacide®, Uroquid®)	50-75 mg/kg/24 h in 4 divided doses (O) Adult: 1 gm q 6 h (O)	Tablets: 0.35, 0.5, 1 gm Granules: 0.5, 1 gm Suspension: 250, 500 mg/5 ml
Metronidazole (Flagyl®)	15-35 mg/kg/24 h q 8 h in divided doses (O) Adult: 250 mg q 8 1 (O)	Tablets: 250 mg
Minocycline HCL (Minocin®)	4 mg/kg/24 h q 12 h in divided doses (O) Adult: 100 mg q 12 h (O)	Capsules: 50, 100 mg Syrup: 50 mg/5 ml

Monostat-Derm® (miconazole nitrate)	Apply 3 times a day to affected area	Cream (2 percent): 1/2, 1, and 3 oz tubes
Moxalactum disodium (Moxam®)	50-200 mg/kg/24 h q 6 h in divided doses (IV) Adult: 2-6 gm/24 h (IV)	Vials: 1, 2 gm in 10 or 20 ml
Nafcillin monohydrate, sodium (Nafcil®, Unipen®)	50-100 mg/kg/24 h q 6 h in divided doses (O) Max: 2-3 gm/24 h (O) 150 mg/kg/24 h q 6 h in divided doses (IM, IV) Max: 8-10 gm/24 h (IV)	Capsules: 0.25, 0.5, 1 gm Solution: 250 mg/5 ml Vial: 0.5, 1, and 2 gm
Nalidixic acid (NeGram®)	55 mg/kg/24 h q 6 h in divided doses (O) Adult: 1 gm q 6 h (O)	Tablets: 0.25, 0.5, and 1 gm Suspension: 250 mg/5 ml
Nitrofurantoin (Furdantin®, Nitrex®)	5-7 mg/kg/24 h q 6 h in divided doses (O) Adult: 50-100 mg q 6 h (O)	Tablets: 50, 100 mg Suspension: 25 mg/5 ml
Nitrofurantoin macrocrystals (Macrofurantin®)	5-7 mg/kg/day q 6 h in divided doses (O) Adult: 50-100 mg q 6 h (O)	Capsules: 25, 50, and 100 mg
Nystatin (Mycostatin®, Nilstat®)	4-6 ml/dose or 1 tab/dose q 6 h (O)	Suspension: 100,000 U/ml Tablets: 500,000 U
Oxacillin, sodium (Bactocill®, Prostaphlin®)	50-100 mg/kg/24 h q 6 h in divided doses (O) Max: 2-3 gm/24 h (O) 100-200 mg/kg/24 h q 6 h in divided doses (IV, IM) Max: 8-10 gm/24 h (IV)	Capsules: 250, 500 mg Solution: 250 mg/5 ml Vial: 0.25, 0.5, 1, 2, and 4 gm
Oxytetracycline	25-50 mg/kg/24 h q 6 h in divided doses (O) Max: 2-3 gm/24 h (O)	Capsules: 250 mg
Oxytetracycline, calcium	25-50 mg/kg/24 h q 6 h in divided doses (O) Max: 2-3 gm/24 h (O)	Syrup: 125 mg/5 ml
Oxytetracycline HCL (Terramycin®)	25-50 mg/kg/24 h q 6 h in divided doses (O) Max: 2-3 gm/24 h (O)	Capsules: 125, 250 mg

CHEMOTHERAPEUTIC DRUGS (continued)

Penicillin G, benzathine (Bicillin®)	50,000 units/kg—1 dose (IM)	Vial: 3 million units Vial: Equal parts of procain penicillin G and benzathine Vial: 3:1 parts of benzathine and procaine penicillin G
Penicillin G, potassium (Pentids®, Pfizerpen G®, Penicillin G® potassium, S-K Penicillin G®)	25-50 mg/kg/24 h q 6-8 h in divided doses (O) Max: 2-3 gm/24 h (O) 50,000-250,000 units/kg/24 h q 4 h in divided doses (IM, IV)	Tablets: 125, 150, 250, and 500 mg Syrup: 125, 250, 500 mg/5 ml Vial: 1, 2, 10, and 20 million units
Penicillin G, procaine (Crysticillin®, Duracillin®, Wycillin®)	25,000-50,000 units/kg/24 h q 12-24 h in divided doses (IM)	Vial: 0.3, 0.6, 1.2, and 2.4 million units
Penicillin G, sodium (Sodium Penicillin G®)	50,000-250,000 units/kg/24 h q 2-6 h (IM, IV) Max: 20 million units/24 h (IV)	Vial: 5 million units
Penicillin V (Betapen-VK®, Ledercillin VK®, Pen Vee K®, Pfizerpen VK®, Robicillin VK®, SK Penicillin VK®, Uticillin VK®, V-Cillin-K®, Vestids®)	25-50 mg/kg/24 h q 6-8 h in divided doses (O) Max: 2-3 gm/24 h (O)	Tablets: 125, 250, and 500 mg Solution: 125, 250 mg/5 ml Drops: 125, 250 mg/5 ml
Piperazine citrate (Antepar®)	75 mg/kg/24 h q 24 h (O) Max: 3.5 gm/24 h (O)	Tablets (wafer): 500 mg Syrup: 500 mg/5 ml
Polysporin® ointment	Apply to affected area 2-3 times a day	10,000 units polymyxin B sulfate and 500 units bacitracin zinc per gm 15, 30 gm tubes
Pyrantel (Antiminth®)	11 mg/dose [1 dose (O)] Max: 1 gm/24 h	Suspension: 250 mg/5 ml
Pyrvinium pamoate (Povan®)	5 mg/kg, 1 dose (O) Max: 7 tablets (O)	Tablets: 50 mg
Rifampin (Rifadin®, Rimactane®)	10-20 mg/kg/24 h q 12 h in divided doses (O) Max: 600 mg/24 h (O)	Capsules: 300 mg

Drug	Dose	Supply
Streptomycin sulfate (Streptomycin®)	20-30 mg/kg/24 h q 12 h in divided doses (IM) Max: 1-2 gm/24 h (IM)	Vial: 1, 5 gm
Sulfadiazine	120-150 mg/kg/24 h q 4-6 h in divided doses (O)	Tablets: 0.3, 0.5 gm
Sulfasiazine sodium (Sulfadiazine®)	100 mg/kg/24 h q 6-8 h in divided doses (SC, IV)	Ampules: 2.5 gm
Sulfamethizole (Proklar®, Sulfadyne®, Thiosulfil®)	30-45 mg/kg/24 h q 6 h in divided doses (O) Adult: 0.5-1.0 gm q 6-8 h (O)	Tablets: 0.25, 0.5 gm Suspension: 0.25 gm/5 ml
Sulfamethoxazole (Gantanol®)	50-60 mg/kg/24 h q 12 h in divided doses (O) Adult: 2 gm stat and 1 gm q 8 h (O)	Tablets: 0.5 gm Suspension: 0.5 gm/5 ml
Sulfasalazine (Azulfidine®, SAS-500®)	30-60 mg/kg/24 h q 4-8 h (O) Max: 3-4 gm/24 h (O)	Tablets: 500 mg
Sulfisoxazole (Gantrisin®, SK Soxazole®)	120-150 mg/kg/24 h q 4-6 h in divided doses (O) Max: 4-6 gm/24 h (O)	Tablets: 0.5 gm Syrup or Suspension: 0.5 gm/5 ml
Sulfisoxazole, acetyl (Lipo-Gantrisin®)	120-150 mg/kg/24 h q 12 h in divided doses (O) Max: 4-6 gm/24 h (O)	Suspension: 1 gm/5 ml
Sulfisoxazole, diolamine (Gantrisin®)	100 mg/kg/24 h q 6-8 h in divided doses (SC, IV)	Vial: 2 gm
Tetracycline (Achromycin®, Cyclopar®, Panmycin®, Retet®, Robitet®, S-K Tetracycline®, Samycin®, Tetracycline®, Tetracyn®, Tetrex®)	25-50 mg/kg/24 h q 6 h in divided doses (O) Max: 2-3 gm/24 h (O)	Capsules: 250, 500 mg Syrup: 125 mg/5 ml Suspension: 125, 250 mg/5 ml
Thiabendazole (Mintezol®)	50 mg/kg/24 h q 12 h in divided doses (O)	Tablets (chewable): 500 mg Suspension: 500 mg/5 ml

CHEMOTHERAPEUTIC DRUGS (continued)

Drug	Dosage	Supply
Trimethoprim (Prolorprim®, Trimpex®)	4 mg/kg/24 h q 12 h in divided doses (O) (Not approved for children under 12 yrs of age.)	Tablets: 100 mg
Trimethoprim (TMP)-Sulfamethoxazole (SMX) (Bactrim®, Septra®)	6-12 mg TMP/30-60 mg SMX/kg/24 h q 12 h in divided doses (O)	Tablets: 80 mg TMP/400 mg SMX Tablets: 160 mg TMP/800 mg SMX Suspension: 40 mg TMP/200 mg SMX/5 ml
Trisulfapyrimidines (Terfonyl®, Neotrizine®)	120-150 mg/kg/24 h q 4-6 h in divided doses (O) Max: 4-6 gm/24 h (O)	Tablets: 0.5 gm Suspension: 125 mg/5 ml
Vancomycin HCL (Vancocin®)	40 mg/kg/24 h q 6 h in divided doses (IV) Max: 2-4 gm/24 h (IV)	Bottle: 10 gm Vial: 500 mg

STEROIDS

Drug	Dosage	Supply
Cortisone acetate	General use: Dosage varies with patient, disease and response (O, IM)	Tablets: 5, 10, and 25 mg Injection: 25, 50 mg/ml
Depo-Medrol® (methylprednisolone acetate)	Repository injection 20-80 mg/ml (IM)	Vial: 1, 5 ml
Hydrocortisone	4/5 cortisone dose (O, IM, IV)	Tablets: 5, 10, and 20 mg Oral suspension: 10 mg/5 ml Ophthalmic suspension: 0.5-2.5 percent Topical: 1 percent Vial: For dilution IV: 2 ml vials 100 mg/ml and 100 mg/20 ml Vial: For IM: 5 ml vials 50 mg/ml Intra-articular: 5 ml vials 20-50 mg/5 ml
Hydrocortisone sodium succinate (Solu-Cortef®)	Dosage: Varies from 20-240 mg/daily depending on the disease being treated	Vial: 100, 250, 500, and 1,000 mg/vial

Drug	Dosage	Form
Prednisone	2 mg/kg 24 h every 6-8 h Dosage: 5-60 mg/24 h depending upon specific disease (O)	Tablets: 1, 2.5, 5, 10, 20, and 50 mg
Triamcinolone (Aristocort®)	Initial: 0.5 mg/kg/24 h Maintenance: 0.1 mg/kg/24 h Divide 24 h dose into 4 equal doses (O)	Tablets: 1, 2, 4, and 8 mg

MISCELLANEOUS DRUGS

Drug	Dosage	Form
Alupent® (Metaproterenol sulfate)	6-9 yrs, 10 mg 3-4 times/24 h (O) 9 yrs and over 20 mg 3-4 times/24 h (O)	Tablets: 10, 20 mg Syrup: 10 mg/5 ml
Atropine sulfate	0.01-0.02 mg/kg/dose Max: 0.4 mg (SC)	Vial: 0.4 mg (1/150 grain)/1 ml
Belladona tincture	0.1 ml/kg/24 h Not to exceed 3.5 ml/24 h Divide into 3 doses (O)	Tincture (USP): 1 ml—about 0.3 mg of atropine (1/200 grain)
Dramamine® (Dimenhydrinate)	5 mg/kg/24 h Children 8-12 yrs: 25-50 mg (O) Adult: 50 mg (O) Max: 150 mg/24 h divided into 4 doses (O, R, IM)	Tablets: 50 mg Suppositories: 100 mg Liquid: 12.5 mg/4 ml Ampules: 50 mg/ml
Eucerin®	Apply 2-3 times a day to affected area	1 lb (50 percent water in oil emulsion of petrolatum, mineral oil, mineral wax, and wave wax alcohols)

Gamma globulin
(immune globulin)
	Hypogammaglobulinemia:
	  1.2 ml/kg initially then 0.66 ml/kg
	  (0.30 ml/lb) q 3-4 wks (IM)
	Measles:
	  Preventive dose: 0.25 ml/kg
	  Attenuation: 0.05 ml/kg (IM only)
	Hepatitis:
	  Preventive dose: Hepatitis A
	                        Hepatitis B
	                        (See Appendix I)
	Specific Hepatitis immune globulin
		16 percent solution USP

MISCELLANEOUS DRUGS *continued*

Drug	Dose	Supply
Gantrisin Ophthalmic®	Solution: 4 percent: 1-2 drops each eye q 2 h initially, decrease to 4 times/24 h	15 ml
Ipecac syrup	Emetic dose: 5-10 ml (O) Repeat in 20-30 min if needed	Syrup USP
Lubriderm®	Apply 2-3 times a day to affected area	Cream: 45, 120 gm Oil bath: 240 ml
Magnesium hydroxide (Milk of Magnesia®)	Cathartic: 0.5 ml/kg/dose (O)	USP magna
Magnesium sulfate (Epsom salt)	Cathartic: 0.25 gm/kg/dose (O)	Ampules: 50 percent
Naphcon-A® ophthalmic	Solution: 0.025 percent naphazoline HCL and 0.3 percent pheniramine maleate 1-2 drops each eye 2-3 times daily	15 ml
Thorazine® (chlorpromazine)	2.0 mg/kg/24 h Adult: 10-25 mg divided into 3-4 doses (O, IM) Rectal dose: Double above Toxic reactions: Jaundice (reversible)	Tablets: 10, 25, 50, and 100 mg Spansules: 30, 75, 150, and 200 mg Suppositories: 25, 100 mg Ampules: 25, 50 mg
Vasocon-A® ophthalmic	Solution: 0.05 percent naphazoline HCL and 0.05 percent antazoline phosphate 1-2 drops each eye 2-3 times daily	15 ml

References

Nelson, W. E. *Textbook of Pediatrics*, 11th Edition, W. B. Saunders, Philadelphia, 1979.
Facts and Comparisons. *Drug Information* Facts and Comparisons, Inc., St. Louis, Mo., 1981.
Nelson, J. D. *Pocketbook of Pediatric Antimicrobial Therapy,* 4th Edition. Jodone Publishing Co., Dallas, 1981-82.

INDEX

A

Abdominal pain, 35
Abrasions, 74
Acetaminophen, 26, 151
Acetylsalicylic acid, 151
ACTH, 99
Acute external otitis, 68
Acute otitis media, 69
Adenovirus, 71
Adrenalin, 21, 151
Airway, 23
Alcohol, 23
Alcohol, 52
Allergic conjunctivitis, 82
Allergic rhinitis, 82
Alupent®, 22, 164
Amebiasis, 122
Amikacin, 156
Aminophylline, 153
Amoxicillin, 21, 156
Ammonia inhalant, 21
Amphetamine sulfate, 151
Ampicillin, 156
Amytal®, 155
Analgesics, 151
Anaphylaxis, 104
Animal bites, 95
Anorexia nervosa, 47
Anticholinergic alkaloids abuse, 54
Antihistamines, 22, 80-83, 92
Antirabies serum, 98
Antisocial personality, 45
Antivenin
 administration, 97
 composition, 97
 dosage, 97
 reactions, 99
Antivenin package (black widow spider), 23, 99
Ant bites, 79
Anxiety disorders, 41
Appendicitis, acute, 36
Appendix I, 121
Appendix II, 150
Aramine, 22, 150
Aristocort, 164
Arrest, cardiac, 122
Ascariasis, 123
Aspirin, 22, 151
Asthma, 83
Atarax®, 155
Atropine sulfate, 164
Attention deficit disorder, 44
Auralgan, 23

Autism, 61
Avoidant disorder, 42

B

Bacillary dysentery (See Shigellosis), 145
Bacitracin® ointment, 21, 156
Bacterial conjunctivitis, 87
Bacterial pneumonia, 138
Baking soda, 23
Barbiturates abuse, 53
Behavior disorders, 44
Belladonna, tincture, 164
Benadryl®, 22, 153
Benztropine mesylate, 22
Betadine® ointment, 74, 156
Betadine® solution, 23, 156
Bicillin®, 161
Bites
 animal, 95
 centipedes, 100
 gila monster, 101
 insects, 78
 mites, 100
 scorpion, 101
 snake, 90
 spider, 99
 tick, 100
Black widow spider, 99
Blepharitis, 88
Blisters, 75
Blood in urine, 38
Botulism, 129,
Brown spider bite, 100
Bulimia, 48
Burns, 105

C

CPR—Cardiopulmonary resuscitation (see Cardiac arrest, 112), 119
Calamine lotion, 23
Calcium gluconate, 23
Camp standards, 1
Camp nurse license, 5
Camp physician license, 5
Carbenicillin, 157
Carbuncles, 75
Cardiac arrest, 112
Cardiopulmonary resuscitation, 113
Cat scratch fever, 124
Cefaclor, 157
Cefadroxil, 157
Cefotaxime, 157
Centipede bite, 100
Cephalexin, 21

Cephalexin monohydrate, 157
Cephalothin, 157
Cephapirin, 157
Cercariae dermatitis (swimmer's itch), 81
Chalazion, 86
Chemotherapeutic drugs, 156
Chest injuries, 108
Chickenpox, 124
Chigger bite (red bug), 100
Chloral hydrate, 155
Chloramphenicol, 157
Chloromycetin otic solution, 23
Chlor-Trimeton, 22, 153
Choking on food, 110
Chronic otitis media, 71
Clindamycin, 158
Clostridial (food poisoning), 37, 130
Codeine, 22, 151
Cold, common, 125
Colorado tick fever, 123
Coly-mycin S otic solution, 23
Conduct disorder, 45
Conjunctivitis, 82
Constipation, 40
Convulsion, 118
Cortisporin otic suspension, 23
Coxsackie viruses A & B, 128
Criteria for death, 117

D

Daily log, 12
Darvon®, 22, 151
Debrox, 23
Demeclocycline, 158
Demerol, 22, 151
Depression, 49
Desenex ointment, 23
Developmental disorders, 60
Dexedrine® sulfate, 151
Diabetes, 62
Diarrhea, 37
Diazepam, 22
Dicloxacillin, 100, 158
Dilantin®, 155
Dimenhydrinate, 164
Dimetapp®, 154
Diphenhydramine hydrochloride, 153
Diphenylhydantoin sodium, 155
Diphtheria, 125
Dog bites, 96
Doxycycline, 158
Dramamine®, 39, 164
Drowning, 110
Drug abuse, 52
Dysentery, 145
Dyslexia, 60

E

Ear, foreign bodies, 71
Eating disorders, 47
Echo virus, 70, 136
Electrical burns, 113
Emergency room, 11
Emergency tracheotomy, 111
Encephalitis (arthropod-borne viral), 122
Encopresis, 49
Enterobiasis vermicularis, 127
Enterovirus, 127
Enuresis, 48
Ephedrine sulfate, 152
Epilepsy, 52
Epinephrine, 83, 93, 151
Equanil®, 155
Erysipelas, 146
Erythromycin, 78, 158
Eucerin®, 76, 164
Examination forms, 5, 8, 9, 11
Extendryl®, 23, 154
Eye
    blepharitis, 88
    ecchymosis, 85
    fluorescin strip, 85
    foreign body, 85
    hemorrhage, 86
    homatropine, 93
    hordeolum (sty), 86
    laceration, 85

F

Fainting, 39
Fever, 38
Fire setting, 46
First aid kits, trip, 26
Fish hooks (removal of), 32
Food (choking), 110
Food poisoning, 37
Food storage, 2
Foreign bodies
    in ear, 71
    in eye, 85
    in nose, 71
    in skin, 75
Forms
    accident report, 18-19
    health history, 6-7
    female health history, 8
    male health history, 9
    health record, 16
Fracture, 108
Furnuncle, 75

G

Gamma globulin, 164
Gantrisin, 165

Gentimicin, 159
German measles, 143
Gila monster bites, 101
Glucose, 5% in saline, 23
Gonorrhea, 131
Griseofulvin, 159, 170

H

Haemophilus aegyptius, 87
Hallucinogens abuse, 54
Haloperidol, 54
Handicapped child, 57
Haverhill fever (rate bite fever), 139
Head injuries, 108
Headache, 35
Health screening, 3
Heat cramps, 103
Heat exhaustion, 102
Heat stroke (heat retention), 103
Hepatitis, 131
Herpangina, 133
Herpes zoster, 124
Homatropine, 89
Homesickness, 42
Hordeolum (sty), 86
Hospital rooms, 11
Hospitalization records, 11
Hydrocortisone, 22, 95, 163
Hydrogen peroxide, 23
Hyperactivity, 44
Hyperglycemia, 63
Hypoglycemia, 64

I

Imiprimine hydrochloride, 22
Immunization (Schedule for), 31
Immunotherapy, 82
Impetigo contagiosum, 76
Inclusion blennorrhea, 88
Infectious mononucleosis, 133
Influenza, 134
Insect bites, 79
Ipecac syrup, 23, 165
Isuprel, 22, 152

K

Kenalog 10, 22
Keratoconjunctivitis, 87

L

Leptospirosis, 135
Levophed®, 22, 152
Librium, 22
Licensing (nurse/physician), 5
Lidocaine, 22
Loxosceles (brown spider bite), 100

Lubriderm, 23, 165
Luminol®, 155

M

Magnesium hydroxide, 165
Magnesium sulfate, 165
Malpractice, 118
Mania, 50
Marijuana, 53
Measles, 142
Mebendazole, 21, 159
Meningitis, 135
Meperidine, 92
Meprobamate, 155
Metaramine bitartrate, 107, 152
Methacycline, 159
Methenamine, 159
Metronidazole, 159
Milk of Magnesia®, 23, 165
Miltown, 155
Mineral oil, 23
Minocycline, 159
Miscellaneous drugs, 159
Mononucleosis, 133
Monostat-Derm cream, 21, 79, 160
Morphine sulfate, 22, 153
Motion sickness, 39
Moxalactum, 160
Mumps, 136
Mycostatin, 160

N

Nafcillin, 160
Nalidixic acid, 160
Naphcon-A® solution, 87, 165
Neck injuries, 109
Negri bodies, 96
Nembutal®, 155
Neosporin ophthalmic ointment, solution, 21
Neo-Synephrine (in shock), 107
Night terrors, 47
Nightmares, 47
Nitrofurantoin, 160
Normal saline, 23
Nose, foreign bodies, 71
Nosebleed, 68
Nupercainal, 23
Nystatin, 21, 160

O

Otic Demeboro solution®, 23
Otitis externa (swimmer's ear), 68
Otitis media, 69
Overanxious disorder, 43
Oxacillin sodium, 21, 160
Oxtetracycline, 160

P

Panic disorder, 43
Paraldehyde, 155
Parent letters, 14
PBZ®, 23, 154
PCP (Phencyclidine) abuse, 53
Pediculosis (body lice), 39, 136
Penicillin, 21, 161
Penicillin G-benzathine, 21, 161
Penicillin G-procaine, 21, 161
Penicillin V, 21, 161
Pentobarbital sodium, 155
Periactin®, 23, 154
Personnel, 13
Pharyngitis, 154
Pharyngoconjunctival fever, 67
Phenergan® hydrochloride, 154
Phenobarbital, 22, 155
Phobias, 43
Physical examination form (pre-camp), 5, 8, 9, 11
Pica, 48
Pink eye, 87
Pinworm infection (thread worm), 127
Piperazine citrate, 161
Pneumonia, 138
Poison ivy dermatitis, 74
Poliomyelitis, 128
Polysporin ointment, 23, 161
Prednisone, 22, 164
Prep tray, 31
Procyclidine hydrochloride, 22
Promethazine hydrochloride, 154
Psittacosis, 139
Psychosis, acute, 51
Pyrantel, 161
Pyribenzamine®, 154
Pyrvinium, 161

R

Rabies, 96
Rat bite fever (Haverhill fever), 139
Reading disorder, 60
Rectal bleeding, 38
Respiratory infections, 67
Resuscitation methods, 113
Rhinitis, allergic, 82
Rifampin, 161
Ringworm, 140
Rocky Mountain spotted fever, 142
Rubella (German measles), 143
Rubeola (measles), 143

S

Saline, 23
Salmonella, 130
Scabies, 144
Scorpion bite, 101
Secobarbital, 156
Sedatives and anticonvulsants, 155
Seizures (convulsion), 59
Separation anxiety disorder, 42
Serum reaction (sensitivity testing for), 93
Sexual "acting out", 46
Shigellosis, 145
Shingles, 124
Shock, 106
Sleep disorder, 46
Sleep terror, 47
Sleepwalking, 46
Snake venom, 90
Snakebite, 91
Sodium bicarbonate, 23
Spider bites, 99
Spinal cord injuries, 109
Sprains, 32
Standards, ACA, 1
Stealing, 45
Stimulants abuse, 68
Stomach ache, 36
Strains, 36
Streptococcal infections, 145
Streptomycin sulfate, 173
Sty (hordeolum), 86
Substance abuse, 52
Sunburn, 73
Sunstroke (heat exhaustion), 102
Swimmer's ear (otitis externa), 68
Swimmer's itch (cercariae dermatitis), 81
Syncope due to heat, 102

T

Tarantula bites, 100
Teldrin®, 154
Terpin hydrate with codeine (cough mixture) 22
Tetanus antitoxin, 32
Tetracycline, 162
Theophylline, 163
Thiabendazole, 162
Tick and mite bites, 79
Tincture of benzoin, 24
Tinea pedis (athlete's foot), 78
Tooth, chipped, 39
Tracheotomy (emergency), 111
Trimethoprim, 163
Trimethoprim-sulfamethoxazole, 163
Tripper's first-aid kit, 26
Tuberculosis, 147
Tularemia, 148

U

Urticaria, 77

V

Ventricular fibrillation, 117
Vernal conjunctivitis, 88
Verrucae (warts), 77
Vomiting, 36

W

Warts (verrucae), 77
Whiplash injury, 110
Whooping cough (pertussis), 137

DATE DUE

DEMCO 38-297